Balancing Act

Memoir of a Southern Woman Doctor

Martha Dukes Yow, M.D.

EAKIN PRESS ☆ Austin, Texas

FIRST EDITION

Published in the United States of America
By Eakin Press
An Imprint of Sunbelt Media, Inc.
Austin, Texas

1-57168-160-4

For my granddaughters:

Megan Keefe and Katy Yow

Contents

Foreword

Dr. Martha Dukes Yow has written a calm and poignant description of her remarkable career in medicine. She entered the Medical College of South Carolina in 1941, four years before Harvard had admitted any women to study medicine. In the years preceding World War II, there were few medical schools in the United States accepting women. This is a fact easilyforgotten in 1997, when one-third to one-half of medical school classes are composed of women. Because of pioneers like Dr. Yow, it is now generally accepted that women are equally as capable of the study and practice of medicine as their male counterparts and equal access of entry into education for the profession of medicine has been achieved.

Dr. Yow's internal strengths and her need to develop and fulfill a sense of self are evident throughout. Her pursuit of personal goals in the face of tradition, especially the tradition of a southern woman, and against accepted family norms, is admirable. We are privileged that she has chosen to share her story with us. It is a valuable and enjoyable saga.

The book describes with good humor the life of a woman medical student and resident living in cramped, makeshift quarters, conditions which were not to change substantially for the next three or four decades. Dr. Yow tells of problems which were neither recognized nor rectified by most institutions, but which potentially compromised the ability of women to function effectively in medical school and post-graduate training positions.

There are no complaints in this book, but rather lessons to be learned from an admired mentor. She taught her students, residents, fellows, and peers lessons about the basic pathogenesis, individual management, and public health measures necessary for several infectious diseases of major significance to children. One need not read her curriculum vitae to be overwhelmed by her accomplishments. She became a fully tenured professor of pediatrics, microbiology, and immunology, and directed the Pediatric Infectious Diseases training program at Baylor College of Medicine for eighteen years. Under her guidance, this program became one of the premier sites for infectious disease training in the United States and, indeed, in the world. She served on the Board of Scientific Counselors for the National Institute of Allergy and Infectious Diseases and she chaired the Infectious Diseases Committee of the American Academy of Pediatrics for two years. The latter group establishes national policy and guidelines for the treatment and prevention of infectious diseases in children in the United States. Dr. Yow's leadership set the standard for all those who have followed in her footsteps.

On numerous occasions, Dr. Yow has been honored for her service to the community, her teaching abilities, and her research. She received the Distinguished Physician award of the Pediatric Infectious Diseases Society and she served for five years as Editor of The Journal of Infectious Diseases, which is the most highly regarded publication in this field in the United States. Her abilities and recognition in this capacity are legendary as she guided the selection of published science in her knowledgeable, but firm gentle fashion.

One would be remiss not to mention that the career of this remarkable woman physician progressed in the face of considerable personal hardship. Happily married and raising her children, as well as functioning in her professional capacity, she became the solid bulwark of her household when her husband contracted an illness which ultimately proved fatal. The strength evidenced by Dr. Yow serves to inspire all of us, and her solutions to the continuing challenges presented by a complex personal and professional life are worth recording and reading. While we celebrate the accomplishments of this extraordinary woman and respect all she has contributed to her family, friends, and medicine, we also look to the future for continued progress in opportunities for similarly outstanding women in the field of medicine.

Catherine M. Wilfert, M.D.
Professor of Pediatrics and Microbiology
Duke University Medical Center

Samuel L. Katz, M.D.
Wilburt C. Davison Professor of Pediatrics
Duke University Medical Center

Preface

Why would I write a book about my life? I'm not an entrepreneur, a movie star, or a first lady. I'm a retired woman physician and professor, a wife, mother, and grandmother, and I first conceived of writing a story of my life for my granddaughters. In my busy life, I had little opportunity to tell them stories about my childhood or about their Southern heritage. Now, at seventy, I'm retired, a decision necessitated by old bones and joints, and living in California where my husband had always dreamed of retiring. So here, overlooking the hills and canyons of Southern California, missing medicine and missing Texas where I had lived for forty years, I started this book as an antidote for homesickness.

I would tell my granddaughters about growing up in a small town in the deep South, the challenge of medical school, and the fun of being one of two girls in a class of forty-four boys. I would tell them, too, about the vicissitudes of establishing myself in the male arena of academic medicine, and the difficulties of balancing home and career. Most of all, though, I wanted them to know of the intense gratification I experienced as a doctor and I wanted them to hear how exciting, rewarding, and challenging my life has been because of my choice to be a wife and mother as well as a doctor. I hoped to inspire them, I think, to work toward the fulfillment of their own dreams.

Then the idea for the book began to change. Young women doctors to whom I had served as a mentor had always expressed interest in my stories and had asked me what it was like to be a woman doctor thirty, forty, or fifty years ago. They had urged me to record some of my experiences and ideas about women in medicine. As I thought about this audience, my thoughts shaped themselves in a different way. I began to recall the tremendous change in attitudes toward women doctors over the last fifty years, but I also saw women in medicine today oftentimes struggling with the same issues that I faced as a young wife and mother. I realized that the women of today pursuing medicine as a career still face many difficult choices as they try to define themselves in their careers and also seek to live full, gratifying personal lives.

Finally, the book became a chronicle for other young working women, not in medicine, who heard me give informal lectures about combining a career and family. These women encouraged me to broaden the scope of the book to encompass experiences common to all career women.

Writing the book has been fun and has helped me to phase into a new life style. I hope that it will give other women, involved in their own balancing acts, encouragement and enjoyment.

Acknowledgments

I thank my family and friends for the support and encouragement they gave me while I was writing this journey through time. They helped me reconstruct and verify my memories, and it has been a valuable opportunity to renew old friendships and to strengthen old ties. I express especial appreciation to Roseland Klein for her expert editorial assistance and her humor and understanding of Southern attitudes; to Adrian Balch for typing and retyping the many versions of the book and her many trips to the medical library; to Elizabeth Waters, Executive Director of Alumni Affairs of The Medical University of South Carolina, who helped me locate historical information about the medical school and about women in medicine; and to my husband, Bob Roessler, a Yankee, who encouraged me to record these memories, saying that Southerners must have a special gene for story telling and hyperbole.

Chapter 1

My Southern Childhood

My earliest memories, which begin in 1926 when I was four years old, are warm and happy. There is no continuum to them; they are just a series of vignettes. I remember one street of the old low country South Carolina town of Hampton, one house, and one small store. The street was unpaved, the sidewalk a wonderful white beach-like sand, and the store a small room with kegs and open bags of rice and other staples. To the right of the entrance a slanted front glass case held a wealth of jaw breakers, all-day suckers, candy watermelon slices, small wax vials filled with a pink sweet liquid, candy shaped like bananas, candy canes, and licorice sticks. Memories of the street and the store fuse because I was allowed to walk alone the short half block from home to the store. I always wanted to prolong the pleasure of spending my penny, so on the way I would stoop down, make a sandy mound, hide the penny, and then search for it. There was always a heart-stopping moment when I thought I'd truly lost it.

When I'd arrive at the store, the storekeeper seemed to have unlimited time to let me decide between a jawbreaker or an all-day sucker – my usual choices because they lasted longer than the other candies. Jawbreakers were best, but concern for my teeth always brought the admonition from my mother, "Suck it, don't chew it." So, for an hour or so, the jawbreaker's sweetness would diffuse slowly and delectably in my mouth.

Another early image of South Carolina is of my father coming down the sidewalk toward home. I can see him, dapper in blue serge and felt hat in the winter, and Palm Beach whites and a flat-topped straw hat in the summer. With a gush of love, I rushed to meet him and flung myself around his knees. He hugged me and the next part of the ritual was the exploration of his coat pockets to find the small treasures he brought – a piece of candy, gum, or maybe a mouth organ, a top, or some other small toy. This ritual seemed to bring as much joy to my father as to me.

We lived in a frame house with a wide porch across the front. It was close enough to the sandy sidewalk that we could talk with people passing by. In my mind's eye, the porch always has people on it, mostly high school students, friends of my older brother and sister – sitting in rocking chairs, in the swing, or on the porch railing. My brother, Arthur Dow, is wearing white pants and my sister, Catherine, the short flapper skirts of the twenties, her hair in spit curls. Through the screen door and out of the shadowy living room comes tinny music, "Yes sir, she's my baby, No sir, don't mean maybe,Yes sir, she's my baby now. She's got eyes of blue, and I never cared for eyes of blue, but she's got eyes of blue and she's my baby nowww!" Then the group moves into the living room, the thick record platter is turned over, the Victrola is wound, and the group dances the Charleston. Music always formed a background for our lives. Arthur Dow and Catherine competed in the music memory contests conducted in South Carolina at that time, and I frequently was assigned the role of changing the records and keeping the Victrola wound. My ability to identify classical music now is very poor, but I always recognize themes from *Carmen*, *La Traviata*, and *The Marriage of Figaro*. I can still hear my sister playing "March Militaire," "Country Gardens," and "Traumerei" on the piano, and hear my brother's deep baritone voice singing "Beautiful Dreamer," "I'll Take You Home Again, Kathleen," and "The Bonny Bonny Banks o' Loch Lomond."

Other memories of these early years bring back my maternal grandparent's home in Greenwood, a large mill and railroad town in the Piedmont of South Carolina. We felt very close to Mother's large, extended family with whom we spent many summers. In the 1920s, Greenwood was a metropolis of 15, 000, with tree-lined streets and sidewalks, a movie theater, a busy train station, numerous stores, and most importantly, an ice cream parlor called the Kandy Kitchen. Summer there felt cool, fresh, and crisp after the heat and humidity of the low country and my grandparents' house was light and airy. My grandfather played games with me, took me for walks, and told me stories about his experiences as a Confederate soldier as he showed me the sepia pictures in an old Civil War album.

When I was five, both of my grandparents died and my Aunt Lala became my substitute grandmother. Lala, or "La" as the nieces and nephews called her, permeates my Greenwood memories. Lala was a quiet, sweet, but brisk little lady who always wore dainty, crisp cotton frocks printed with small delicate flowers, and in the mornings, these were covered by fresh starched aprons. She loved children and seemed intuitively to know what they would enjoy. She and Uncle Morehead married late in life and lived with my grandparents. They never had any children of their own, so Lala enjoyed all the nieces and nephews. I was her special favorite, and later I found that she had asked to adopt me when Mother and Daddy were having severe financial problems. Her request was not considered seriously, but throughout my childhood, I always knew she loved me and I could count on her.

I visited her in the summers and I could depend on receiving boxes of surprises from her all during the year. She seemed to know just what a child would like, wrapping small boxes individually so I had the pleasure of opening up a box and finding several separately wrapped gifts such as a new dress, a set of jacks, card games, a tea set, and once a tiny electric marshmallow grill. Each time when I arrived in Greenwood, she had all the issues of *Pictorial Review*, a popular women's magazine at that time, saved so that I could cut out the monthly pages of Dolly Dimple Clothes for my paper doll. Later I found out that she'd lend Mother money at Christmas so that Santa Claus could leave the expected presents. Although Lala was a very responsible adult, she played with me as if she herself were a joyful child.

It was fun to watch Lala run the house. Right after breakfast she went out to cut flowers still fresh with dew before the sun would make them wilt. Lala had a green thumb and grew beautiful dahlias, cosmos, snapdragons, and chrysanthemums. Flowers arranged, she proceeded to the marketing by telephone, of course: "Hello, Central, give me Mason's Grocery Store. Hello, Mr. Mason. This is Mrs. Morehead." Then they exchanged a few pleasantries before they dealt with her order. "How are the cantaloupes, today? Well, I'll take two, and two pounds of onions and, please, grind me some nice lean beef, about a pound and a half." And so they went through the list, item by item. Later in the day, the grocery boy would come up the back steps and deposit the bags on the kitchen table. Meantime, two other important matters had been handled. The ice card had been put in the window with the 25-pound label pointing upward. The card was reversible and the iceman knew the amount requested by which side was visible and which end was up. When he arrived in his horse drawn wagon, I was allowed to go out to ask for ice chips that fell as he sawed off the 25-pound block and set his tongs in it. After he deposited the ice in the icebox, we began to listen for the vegetable wagon. Then both Lala and I went out to the street to select fruits and vegetables – string beans, lima beans, apples, tomatoes, blackberries, huckleberries. The berries were measured in pint- and quart-sized worn coffee cans and the vegetables were weighed on a rusty scale hanging from the support of the canopy that protected the produce from the sun.

Now, with all the supplies laid in, we sat at the kitchen table or in rocking chairs and snapped beans, shelled peas, or peeled apples for pie. This was a companionable time, and if the aunts or other cousins were present, a time for good conversation.

When evening arrived, the adults would gather on the porch while we played under the street lights or caught fireflies. Later, as we tired, we sat on the steps hearing the creak of the swing and the rhythm of the rocking chairs as the adults talked about community happenings and told funny stories on each other. We were aware of which in-law uncle was a ne'er-do-well, which one exaggerated and always had get-rich-quick schemes, which aunt was sickly, and which was over protective of her children; but the sense of family unity was strong and there was a sense of remarkable tolerance of each other's frailties. Even as children, we knew how the family fit together.

We heard stories of flirty grass widows (divorced women), and those who had just had their hair bobbed, hennaed or marcelled (the forerunner of the permanent). The mothers would tell about plucking up their courage to have their own hair bobbed, walking to the barber shop only to lose their nerve and return home with their long tresses. The fathers were always relieved. We heard about illnesses of relatives and friends and the stories that impressed me most were accounts of the traditional southern lady's traditional malady, the nervous breakdown, or "taking to one's bed" over disappointments, such as breaking up with one's sweetheart. It was all so sad and romantic!

When I visited with Lala and her husband, Uncle Morehead, I stayed in a spacious, cheerful bedroom. The bed linens were beautifully ironed and monogrammed or edged with handmade embroidery or crochet. A pleasant cool breeze usually blew across the bed from the windows on either side, and at night, I heard dogs barking nearby and far out into the country side.

Since Greenwood was a railroad town there were distant train noises in the quiet night. In the morning, I was awakened by roosters' crowing. It seemed to me that they crowed in a regular sequence going out in a great circle and then starting all over again. I always wakened with a sense of excitement. "Where am I? Oh, I'm in Greenwood. I wonder what we'll do today. Maybe I'll skate or we'll go downtown to the Kandy Kitchen, or maybe La will make sassafras tea from the tree outside and we'll have a tea party." My choices seemed endless.

* * * * * * * *

After living in Hampton for two years, my parents moved us to Bowman in Orangeburg County, my father's home territory where three of his six sisters and their families lived. Daddy had grown up on a farm five miles from Bowman and had relatives under every bush. We moved into a house across a sandy street from one aunt and our backyard was separated by our barn from another aunt's and uncle's barn and backyard. I had a total of eleven cousins in that one block.

My father had always uprooted our family every one to two years (my older sister later told me that we had lived in four towns in Georgia, North Carolina, and South Carolina by the time I was six), but when we made this move, my mother put her foot down about the constant changing from place to place. She got a job teaching English and Latin and said Bowman was where we were going to live from now on. Daddy got a teaching job in another town seventy miles away where he spent Monday through Friday and came home for weekends.

Bowman was a farming town located on the main highway, still unpaved in 1927, from Columbia to Charleston. The population was eight hundred, one third white and two thirds black. The stores had the false fronts, popular in the late 1800s, and ran along on either side of the highway for about a half a mile, with houses and two churches lengthening the town to about a mile. A few streets and lanes extended out on either side of the main road. These led to more homes, the grammar school and high school, the grist mill, the cotton gin, and an abandoned brick mill. There was no railroad, no movie theater, no swimming pool.

The town's social life centered around the school and the Baptist and Methodist churches. For women, there was also the missionary society and the U.D.C. (The United Daughters of the Confederacy). The men spent long hours in various stores in town gathered around the pot-bellied stoves, discussing crops, politics, and the all-important weather. Very early, I learned that it either rained too little or too much. If it was dry, the cotton wouldn't bear well. If it was wet, the cotton was big and robust, and the boll weevils were in hog heaven. Also, I learned that an afternoon hail storm could wipe out a farmer's corn crop. Another reality of farm life that children learned very early was the law of supply and demand. If the crop was poor, there was nothing to sell and the prices were high. If the harvest was bountiful, prices were down. Soon, I made up my mind that when I grew up, I didn't want to marry a farmer.

I often think that growing up in a town with limited social life and recreational facilities helped me develop initiative and a vivid imagination. There were few distractions, and there was, of course, no television. The first radio I ever listened to was in one of the grocery stores. The men were gathered round, listening and laughing about how squeaky women's voices sounded on the radio. They stated loudly that women would never have a place in radio.

There were only two telephones in Bowman – one in the doctor's office and one in a home where the living room served as the town's switchboard. The purpose of this latter communication link was, I suppose, to call Orangeburg, the county seat, to arrange for the undertaker or to call the hospital to report incoming emergencies, usually accidents or snake bites. Occasionally, one's distant relatives called "Central" to report serious illness or death, and "Central" had to come to your house to deliver the message. Telegrams, also a very important method of communication in those days, were read in Orangeburg to "Central" in Bowman and "Central" brought the message to you. Despite the lack of telephones, communication within the town was remarkably swift. I never figured it out, but we always knew almost immediately when college boys were in town selling magazine subscriptions, when there was a drummer selling his wares, and when the Fuller Brush salesman was making his rounds.

I used to love it when the man with the brushes would arrive at our door. Mother would invite him into the living room and he would open his suitcase and give an interesting spiel. Finally, mother would order a small bottle of "real vanilla – not artificially flavored vanilla," and then I would get to choose the free gift.

Another way that news traveled in Bowman was via the daily meetings at the post office. The RFD (rural free delivery) postman brought the mail from Orangeburg twice a day and there was much conversation while waiting for his arrival and while opening the individual mailboxes. Various family members alternated in going for the mail, but usually the afternoon pickup was assigned to me.

In the years I lived year round in Bowman, I developed my lifelong love of the South Carolina low country. We lived close to the land. We walked almost everywhere we went and observed all the details of the seasons that one misses riding in cars – the bursting out of wild lilies, violets and dogwood in the spring; the heavy sweet smell of wisteria in the summer; the falling of the red and yellow leaves in the fall; and the beauty of holly trees and Christmas berries, and the deep green and rich clean smell of the long leaf pines on crisp winter days. Daddy took me walking in the swampy woods on the farm where he had grown up and showed me "headache flowers" (wild azaleas), jack-in-the-pulpits, flycatchers, and medicinal herbs around cypress trees with their knobby knees. He talked to me about snakes, raccoons, possums, and about alligator hunts when he was a boy. One night, he took me possum hunting. We didn't see any possums, but we cooked chicken pilau over an open fire and ate mouth-puckering persimmons right off the tree.

If my parents wanted a docile little girl, they must have been disappointed in me. Dolls didn't interest me, and I much preferred climbing trees, playing follow-the-leader, and playing sand lot baseball in the sandy streets beside our houses; but on Sundays, baseball was forbidden, as were cards. On Sundays, we were allowed to play tame games of croquet – boring, boring, boring. The boys didn't like me as a girl, but they sure liked me as a baseball hitter. When they chose up sides and there weren't enough boys, I would be the first girl chosen! I felt like I could hit a ball a country mile and longed to be a boy because I thought the things they got to do were so much more fun and interesting than the games girls wanted to play. I wanted to build things; I hammered and nailed, making play houses I never played in.

I was an energetic, adventurous, determined child and I always seemed to be in trouble, spending hours restricted to the yard as punishment for some misdemeanor. There were many of these, because Mother was very strict and had many rules that I had to break in order to keep up with the gang. By necessity, I became proficient at making up "stories," but somehow, the communications were against me and always, by the time I got home in the afternoon, news of my activities had already reached my mother's ears, and punishment was sure and swift. I spent a lot of time in solitary confinement talking to my dog, who was my constant companion and who shared all my troubles, and looking through our wire fence watching my cousins play. Very early, I was impressed with the importance of either being honest or learning how to lie skillfully in order to save my hide and to avoid retribution. But my worst punishments were always the result of naive lying.

I was called a tomboy, though I hated this label. Mother thought she was reassuring me when she said repeatedly, "Have the courage to be different!" I was different, but how I hated those words. I dreamed of becoming an aviatrix, following in Amelia Earhart's footsteps, or an inventor or discoverer, but at about age eight, I decided I wanted to be a doctor and that never changed.

Life was not all play, though. Arthur Dow, Catherine, and I did a lot of work with few conveniences.My duties included dusting, drying dishes, setting the table, and ironing easy pieces. Each summer morning, I went to the ice house for a block of ice for the refrigerator and pulled it home in my homemade wagon – a hard job on soft, sandy sidewalks. If I stopped for a quick game of hopscotch or marbles, my dawdling was evident by the diminished size of the block of ice. Emptying the drip pan under the ice box was also one of my jobs. Nobody was happier than I when electric refrigerators became available! Less frequent duties were feeding the chickens (which I loathed) and bringing in vegetables from the garden. How okra makes your arms itch!

Occasionally, I had to help wash and hang clothes, but generally, we had a washer woman who boiled the white things in a black iron pot over a fire in the backyard. The clothes were lifted out of the boiling water, using a board bleached by use, and transferred to one of the three galvanized tubs sitting on a bench – one soapy wash on a scrub board and two rinses. All pockets and socks had been turned inside out. When the wash was big, Mother, my sister, and I helped. It took two to wring the sheets and there was an art to getting them on the line without dragging them in the dirt. And, oh, the days when the line broke or when it rained when the clothes were almost dry!

On hot summer mornings, we canned vegetables; we made jam and jelly. You understand I didn't do these things willingly. I was raring to play or to read, but my family believed your work had to be done before you could play. That meant hard work in the mornings because after the big midday meal, few women worked. They took naps, freshened up, and sat on the porch until it was time for a light supper.

After our big dinner came enforced rest time. All little southern girls were supposed to take naps during the heat of the day. That was no hardship for me because, of course, I never napped. I read. I loved to read and read everything I could lay my hands on – books given to me (*Honey Bunch, The Bobbsey Twins, Heidi, Hans Brinker and the Silver Skates, Little Men, Little Women, Jo's Boys*); books I borrowed (Zane Grey and Horatio Alger books, which Mother deplored, but I loved, especially the success stories of the poor struggling boys in *Do or Die* and *Strive and Succeed*). When all these books "suitable to my age" were exhausted, I moved on to my parents' collection – Dickens, Thackeray, the Brontë sisters, Sir Walter Scott, and when I had read them all, I reread them. I cried over *David Copperfield* at least three times. Early in my life, reading became not only a joy, but also an escape I would employ all of my life.

All of my family liked to learn and we did it together at the dining room table. Young families today would be overjoyed by our dining room. They would call it the great room or the den. We used the living room for visitors, for reading, for card playing, and for music, but the dining room was the heart of our home with its big table in the center and rocking chairs around the fireplace. Our house was heated by three fireplaces located in the living room, dining room, and our parents' bedroom. The rest of the house was cold. On winter evenings, the dining room was occupied by all of us, plus the dog and the cat. Mother graded papers or wrote plays for high school performances. Daddy was often away, but when he was there, he usually smoked his pipe and read by the fireplace. There was a cardinal rule – you didn't talk to anyone while he or she was reading or writing. It was quiet, but communal.

The best memory of those evenings is of my bedtime stories. First, there was the mandatory Bible story from Hurlburt's *Story of the Bible*. Mother usually read those to me, but demurred when I wanted always to hear the book of Esther – I loved the romance! Mother insisted on going through the whole Bible sequentially. First things first. Then Daddy and I could get on with our "secular" stories. I would sit on his lap while he shelled pecans or peeled sugar cane for me and told me stories about when he was a boy (he was a wonderful story teller, and my cousins begged him to tell them stories). My second choice, when he didn't want to tell stories, was for him to read *Uncle Remus*, especially the parts where Daddy Jack appears and speaks Gullah. My father spoke Gullah, the dialect of the South Carolina island Negroes, perfectly.

Our first years in Bowman were full and interesting. Catherine and Arthur Dow were in high school, and our house seemed full of lively times piano playing, dancing in the living room, and playing cards. Being the baby, I was on the edge, of course, but often I got to sit in as a fourth at cards. My sister was in charge of me much of the time and sometimes lamented it: "When you grow up and have children I hope they're just as bad as you are!" But her complaints didn't bother me. I knew that, although I was a caboose child, my family loved me.

These happy carefree days came to an abrupt end in 1929 when I was seven. The great depression had hit the country and I became deeply aware of its effect on my family. I didn't understand what it meant when people said the bank had "busted," but I remember my mother crying because our savings were lost and I became acutely anxious about the family's ability to pay the rent and to buy groceries. These were very real concerns. My father lost his job in 1930 and Mother was making only sixty dollars a month. That was what we lived on with the exception of one or two subsequent years when she received a "claim" each month. A claim was a voucher stating that her salary would be paid when the school had the money. Meantime some merchants would cash the claims but charged a high interest rate so our family of five lived on about fifty-five dollars a month for rent, food, insurance premiums, medical care, car payments.

Daddy tried vegetable farming but he didn't make enough to pay his expenses. Even worse than our reduced income was the anxiety that permeated our home about the uncertainty of Mother's having a job. The county school district was out of funds and the school in Bowman was dependent on state funding. Each spring we waited nervously to learn whether the state legislature would approve "state's aid." When it was approved there was a great sense of relief and celebration in the family. Mother had a job for another year!

Despite the pervasive financial insecurity of my childhood, many of my experiences during the depression helped me in later life. I learned a great deal about coping. For example we managed without buying any clothes. After wearing cardboard in our shoes, we learned to resole our shoes ourselves by gluing on rubber soles, and our clothes were remade from handed down clothing from our more affluent cousins. Fortunately, Mother was an accomplished seamstress and often the re-dos were more fashionable than the originals. She was truly inventive and she had a touch of class. She had one sensational creation that all her lady friends coveted. She needed a new hat, so she took a dark red felt hat out of grandmother's old trunk, steamed it, trimmed the brim, turned it around backwards, added a flamboyant ten-cent store plume, wore it at a rakish angle, and created a sensation at church. Living through the depression and understudying my mother certainly taught me to be creative. When you didn't have something, you made it. You learned adaptability. If one approach didn't work, you tried another.

Another important thing I learned during these depression years was responsibility about money matters. By observing my parents, I learned about not incurring debts you couldn't pay, about making arrangements in advance for meeting your obligations, and that once a deal was made, dependability was paramount. Often these deals involved barter. When we didn't have cash, we arranged to pay with fresh vegetables or Mother's famous vegetable soup put up in Mason jars.

Regardless of the accommodations we had to make, we never felt poor. For one thing, complaining was not countenanced in our home; also, everybody was in the same boat. Nobody had any money and many of our neighbors had less than we did. Some people had to be on the dole (acceptance of free flour, sugar, and other food stuffs from the government). Nobody wanted to do this! South Carolinians have fierce pride and a long history of resisting federal interference in their lives, so accepting government handouts was considered a disgrace, but some people had no choice. Recalling some of the abject poverty I observed, I realize that our family was, indeed, not poor. Not only did we have the necessities, but we also were rich in the belief that our straitened circumstances were temporary and that we had good futures.

Hard times or not, there was never any question but that my

brother and sister would go to college, but they knew that they had to do it on their own. My brother entered a statewide competition and won a full, four-year scholarship to the Citadel. He left home in 1929. The next year my sister was off to college on a work scholarship.

Now, at age eight, I was at home alone with my parents and I had to deal with something much worse than the financial difficulties of the depression. I had become old enough to be aware of terrible strife between my parents. I learned later that it had existed throughout their entire marriage but when I was younger I didn't recognize it. Also by then, the tension between them had become much worse and with Arthur Dow and Catherine away from home, Mother and Daddy seemed to give up any semblance of normal family home life. Daddy had screaming jealous rages about Mother's having a job and accused her of causing his failures. The nightly scenes ended with my mother in tears and me too frightened to sleep. I was still too young to understand or to care about the reasons for their incompatibility. I just knew that our home life was miserable. When Daddy took a teaching job in the Florida Everglades, I welcomed the respite from family quarrels.

Away from home, Daddy wrote long, colorful letters describing his life in the Everglades and telling Mother how much he missed her. After a year in Florida, he returned to Bowman. Naively, I thought things would be different between my parents. They were worse. Daddy became angrier and angrier, and Mother became more and more outwardly submissive. My father was fifty-two at the time, and Mother, forty-seven. Now I understand that a form of mental illness had begun to influence my father beyond repair, but then I thought he had just become mean. He began to say horrible things to my mother, accusing her of all sorts of misconduct. At one point, he went to the school board and told them that she was too unstable to teach school. She was subsequently fired. No one challenged Daddy's word so Mother, one of the most respected teachers in Bowman, was out of a job. And although she went to the school board members to try to explain (there was very little knowledge or understanding of mental illness at the time), and begged to be reinstated, they refused.

Mother went to Daddy's family for help in dealing with Daddy, but they thought that she was hysterical and responsible for Daddy's failures. They offered no help. As I sat nervously on the sidelines, a voice in my head began to resound, "I will never get married!"

The summer I was twelve, Daddy became more and more agitated and violent, and Mother and I were forced to leave home. We went to North Carolina to stay with Mother's brother and his wife who were wonderfully kind, but we hated being the "poor relatives" imposing on them. Mother tried to get a teaching job nearby, but as a woman separated from her husband and with only a shaky recommendation from her former school, there was no opportunity for her. After six months, we moved to Savannah to live with my brother, who by now had graduated from college and was working there.

During this time, Daddy was writing sad, repentant letters begging us to come home. Meanwhile, I was begging Mother to get a divorce – I couldn't believe that she even considered going back to my father. In my childish perspective, I didn't take into account two factors: first, to my mother, divorce was a sin; second, divorce was also illegal in South Carolina (incidentally, South Carolina was the last state to legalize divorce and that didn't occur until after World War II) (S.C. Const.).

After a month in Savannah, Mother agreed to go back to Bowman and try again to live with Daddy, but she told him that he would have to provide the living, and he agreed to this arrangement. When we arrived, Daddy was acting much less disturbed and had gotten a government-subsidized job that paid forty dollars a month and he had also begun to truck farm on rented land. But while other people around the nation were singing Roosevelt's song, "Happy Days Are Here Again!," times were still very tough in rural South Carolina. After a year of Daddy's trying to support us, it became clear that Mother needed to supplement the family income and she too got a government job surveying the health needs of the rural poor in our area. The move back to Bowman when I was thirteen was excruciating for me, and I begged my mother up until the last minute not to return. I was afraid of the gossip about my parents and, of course, we were the latest town scandal. Some children said cruel things to me and the young, cliquish girls excluded me. I withdrew.

At first, I could not face school and stayed with my sister, Catherine and her husband. She had married a wonderful man, Rhett Shuler, when I was ten. I stayed with them for about a month. They didn't pressure me about returning to school, and instead were warm and loving. During the day, Rhett took me partridge hunting and taught me to ride horseback and at night, they both played endless games of cards with me. When I finally went back to school, I felt humiliated and disgraced and expressed my feelings by acting arrogant and sarcastic with my classmates and teachers, but somehow, despite my attitude and all the interruptions in schooling, I passed the eighth grade.

Now my self confidence was at an all-time low, I was antagonistic toward my parents, I felt like a misfit in Bowman, and I was very discouraged. But then fate intervened and offered me the opportunity for a more normal life – to live with Lala in Greenwood.

Chapter 2

Leaving Home

IN 1935 WHEN I WAS thirteen, Uncle Morehead died and for the first time in her sixty years, Lala was alone. Terribly lonely, she wrote to Mother and Daddy asking whether I could live with her during the school year. They agreed and I joyfully accepted, welcoming an escape from Bowman and my parents' growing problems.

Since the Depression, Lala had little if any money, so she rented her Greenwood home and leased a small apartment within walking distance of the high school. She, like Mother, had a vein of iron; so instead of complaining about no money, she decided to take in sewing. She was an excellent seamstress and quickly became Greenwood's most sought after dressmaker for fine clothes, supporting the two of us on her earnings.

When I moved to Greenwood, I felt suddenly released from my parents' problems and I made a conscious decision to make a new start and change my attitude – I would study hard, cooperate with my teachers, participate in athletics, and be a real part of the school community. Also, I decided to handle my own problems. In Bowman, Mother had embarrassed me by trying to handle every problem I encountered at school. I hated this intrusion and now I was determined to run my own life. Less consciously, I resisted shouldering anybody else's troubles, so despite Lala's loneliness, I avoided involvement in her problems, such as I had experienced with Mother. My only concession to Lala's needs was to go to church with her on Sunday morning, often on Sunday night, and sometimes, grudgingly, to prayer meeting on Wednesday night. I balked at visiting relatives, a routine Sunday afternoon activity in the deep South.

When I entered the beautiful red brick, colonnaded high school building in September, I began three of the best years of my life. I had left a school of sixty students and entered one of a thousand, a consolidated school of teenagers from the town and the surrounding farms. It was run in a quiet but firm way by the superintendent and by Major Benson, the principal. Major Benson believed in doing things the right way, because it was right. There was no nonsense about it. We were sure that Greenwood High was the best school in South Carolina and that we were there to keep it that way. I cherished the academic reputation and played my heart out in athletics, competing with students from schools all over upper South Carolina. I was in the situation all teenagers need, stability at home and clear-cut rules of behavior at school and in the community.

Since I was a good student, the teachers singled me out for unusual opportunities, including recommending me to the editorial staff of the weekly high school newspaper, *Hi-TYPE*, which became a major part of my life. Athletics were also a big part of my life at Greenwood High. In the fall and winter, I practiced basketball in the big beautiful gymnasium with its light, polished hardwood floors. (In Bowman, the basketball court had been outside and the playing surface was hard dirt, unless it rained, and then it became so muddy that play was impossible.) Basketball was a different game on that wonderful floor. I was never very good at it; although, because of my height (5'8"), I played center on the first team. My speed and agility left something to be desired, but the camaraderie in the afternoons and the excitement of the night games at home and out-of-town competition made me give it my all. From the time I donned that green uniform with the great gold "G" on my bosom, I was a part of the Emerald team from Greenwood High!

If I loved basketball, I was obsessed by tennis. We had outdoor clay courts which were maintained beautifully, and all spring we practiced. I was better at tennis than at basketball, and by my senior year was captain of the team. In both sports, we had wonderful coaches and the competition with teams from other schools was fierce. My English teacher complained that I spent too much time in athletics and too little on academic pursuits, but her complaints did nothing to modify my zest and involvement in sports.

The time in Greenwood was also a time of many wonderful friendships, and I had one "best friend." The day I arrived, a pretty, thin blonde girl appeared on the portico of the magnificent house across the street from the modest house where we lived. She waved and then walked over to introduce herself. Genevieve (Gee) Taylor was one of five sisters being reared by their widowed father. The Taylors were among the wealthiest families in Greenwood, and their home was a white mansion set in a block of tree-shaded green lawn surrounded by a black iron fence. There were porticos with big columns on the front and side, and a circular driveway leading to the side portico. The front entrance was approached by a long brick walk extending across a great green expanse of well-tended lawn. I was to spend many hours in that beautiful house because from the time we met, Gee and I were together every possible minute. Lala became exasperated by the amount of time Gee and I were together, and when apart, we talked on the telephone. Mr. Taylor (Papa) must have had similar feelings about the extra girl who was at his home so much. Gee and I studied together and we talked endlessly. We talked in her living room in front of the fire, in her spacious upstairs bedroom, in the swing on the porch, in the two-way swing on the big front lawn, and as we lingered back and forth across the street between our houses. We never ran out of things to say to each other. We went to the movies about once a week with a group of friends where we were transported by Nelson Eddy and Jeanette McDonald, cried over *Camille*, agonized with Janet Gaynor, and were thrilled by Clark Gable, Fredric March, and Ronald Colman.

Gee was a shy, retiring, romantic, sentimental girl. I, too, was romantic, but with a hard core of realism and a veneer of indifference about boys. We talked endlessly about boys, but were too inhibited to let them know we were interested. We daydreamed about romances where "the man of our dreams" would say, "I adore you. I need you. I can't live without you!" We spent those self-conscious, important, formative years with the loving support of each other.

* * * * * * * *

During my high school years, my mother insisted that I spend my summers in Bowman. And although every morning I would get up with my father and accompany him on his rounds to the farms, there was little real communication between us. At five o'clock in the morning, we went to the tomato field where he supervised the picking and I worked at a tree-shaded, makeshift grading table beside the field. My job was to supervise three black women in grading the tomatoes and "dressing" the crates, which consisted of putting the largest, prettiest tomatoes on top. (This seemed dishonest to me, but I learned that the wholesalers considered it standard practice and they knew that smaller green tomatoes were on the bottom.) It was hot, dirty work, but by late afternoon the crates were ready to go to the farmers' market the next day. Daddy drove a truck the sixty miles to Columbia during the night so that he could arrive in time to get a good spot to have his produce selected by a buyer. It was often disheartening, and sometimes he and the other farmers would bring the fruits and vegetables back and feed them to the hogs rather than accept a price that was too low. When Daddy could afford it, he paid me a dollar or two, and he always gave me the "seconds" to sell door-to-door in Bowman.

The Bowman summers always seemed long, and one summer, out of sheer boredom, I taught myself to type; another summer, I tried to teach myself how to speak French. But mostly, I read and waited to go back to Greenwood and school in the fall. Soon I began to be interested in boys, but was too inhibited to show it. More importantly, they were not interested in me. I was tall, skinny, wore glasses, was arrogant because of insecurity, and talked like an adult. I had no gift for small talk. Occasionally, one of my boy cousins would ask me to go to the movies, always on a double date. He was as socially inept as I was, and as we rode the fifteen miles to Orangeburg, we would sit on the back seat and observe the more glib, sophisticated couple in the front. We didn't have a really great time, but I have always been eternally grateful to him for helping me begin to date. Then from an unexpected source, romance entered my life!

It happened at camp meeting the summer I was fifteen. Each July, the Methodist church held a religious revival at Cattle Creek campground, one of the few remaining old-fashioned religious campgrounds in the United States, on land that my father's family lent to the Methodist church. It was a large, round clearing, about a quarter of a mile in circumference, in a forest of pines and moss-draped oaks. Around the edges of the clearing, permanent "tents" were built, two-story unpainted tin-roofed frame houses that looked like tobacco barns. Each tent had a shed-roofed porch in front with room for rocking chairs and wooden benches on the sides and front for additional seating. The tents sat flat on the ground and the floors downstairs and on the porch consisted of hard-packed dirt covered each year with fresh straw. The main room was used for eating and contained a large plank table and side benches, seating as many as 16 to 20 people. At one end of this front room, rustic stairs led to the two dormitory rooms upstairs – one for men and boys, and one for the female sex. The windows were open slots under the eaves. There was no indoor kitchen. Cooking, a major activity of camp meeting, was carried out in an open shed behind the tent.

The tents were owned by individual families, and each year, the week before camp meeting, there was a flurry of activity. Old straw was swept out, a search for resident snakes conducted, cobwebs brushed off the ceiling, mattresses brought from home and laid side by side on the long platforms built under the windows, firewood stacked by the big outdoor iron stoves, and at the homes of the "tenters" a vast amount of food was prepared to be transported to the campground – hams, pies, cakes.

There were about 25 or 30 tents, but many more than 25 to 30 families attended. The tents were filled with relatives and friends. One tent was exclusively for the Methodist ministers. There were usually 10 or 12 ministers tenting, and on Sunday, the presiding elder for the district would come to preach. The

Methodist women took turns making sure the preachers' tent was bursting with food.

People came from miles around to spend the day and to attend the religious services that were held three times a day – morning, afternoon, and evening. It was not unusual for a family who was tenting to serve midday or evening dinner to 50 or 100 people. It was a great source of pride to be able to say you had 100 people for dinner. Meals were held in shifts – first, second, and third tables.

At one curve of the big clearing stood a simple, small white church and an old cemetery where many of my paternal ancestors were buried. But this was not where camp meeting services were held. They were held in the big, open tin-roofed tabernacle in the center of the campground. Three times a day services were announced by a man blowing on an ancient cow horn. "Hoo, hoo, hoo" – first warning to get quiet and promenaders to assemble in the tabernacle, or to withdraw to porches. Five minutes later, "Hoo, hoo, hoo"– services were to begin. Now it was remarkably quiet except for the minister's voice, the "amens" from the preachers on the left side benches, and the sounds of the grand old hymns.

Promenading at camp meeting was a courting ritual. When we arrived at camp meeting early in the week, the first thing the teenagers did was to go into the woods and cut themselves a walking cane. We chose a small branch or stick about two and a half feet in length and with bark that would slip easily. On this stick, we made elaborate designs in the bark, using pocket knives. Next, we found sturdy vines, wove them into round handles and attached them to our cane, sometimes we left our beautiful canes bare without handles. There were always boys who found "devils' walking canes." These were sticks covered by large thorns. Now with our canes, we were ready to promenade. Groups of girls and groups of boys walked around and around in the big space between the tents and tabernacle, the girls and boys circling in opposite directions so that once in every circle they passed each other face to face.

One by one, boys would screw up their courage, extend their canes and say to the girl of their choice, "You wanna promenade?" If a girl reached out to their canes, she signified acquiescence. Gradually, the separate groups grew smaller and smaller, and twosomes were walking together, often arm-in-arm trying desperately to know what to say to each other. The older generation sat on the porches loosely chaperoning and commenting, "Look, George is promenading with Sarah," or "For goodness sake, when is Ben going to ask Mary Lou to walk with him?" Girls could flirt and signify their enthusiasm to be invited, but only the boys could make the first overture. Some couples became partners for the week; others continued to play the field.

I was not very popular, so I might do a lot of walking before being invited to promenade. Being tall, wearing glasses and looking older than my real age were special handicaps. I suffered agonies of shyness, which didn't emerge as modest ladylike behavior, but came out as arrogance and indifference. Many years later when I had been married twice, one of my old male acquaintances from Bowman said, "If you were interested in boys, why didn't you let us know?"

Then one night when I was fifteen, the unbelievable happened. I was sitting in the choir with my girlfriends (the choir sat on wooden benches on the raised platform behind the pulpit). Someone behind me tapped me on the shoulder and handed me a note. It said, "I'm Sidney Crumpton. Will you promenade with me after the service?" I turned around slightly and saw a man who looked about twenty-five nodding at me. I turned back around, heart pounding, but decided to take a chance; I nodded back, "yes." After the service, we began walking arm-in-arm around and around. Fortunately, we were sheltered from too many prying eyes because of the darkness. There were no electric lights at the campground. Light was afforded by blazing pinewood on layers of sand placed on wooden stands six- to eight-feet square and about six feet off the ground. These "stands" were situated at intervals around the circle in the promenading area.

It was a magical night. The fires flickered on the stands, the moon rose mistily from behind the forest and shone on the moss-festooned oaks spaced here and there throughout the clearing. We walked and we talked. How we talked! Here was somebody who didn't mind my being tall, serious, and sounding like an adult. When he discovered my age, he was somewhat taken aback. He'd thought I was much older when he had passed me the note, but that didn't stop our flow of congeniality. He was a teacher in Greenville, about 100 miles away. This was his first experience at camp meeting and he was enchanted by it. He was teaching until he could save enough to go to divinity school, and in the summers made money traveling around the state recruiting students for the Methodist College, Wofford. He had gone to Wofford himself as had my father, a fact that didn't hurt me when I had to convince my mother that it was safe for me to go out with him in the daytime.

Even the darkness couldn't keep the people on the porches from catching glimpses of us in the firelight and commenting, I'm sure, "Look at Martha Dukes walking with that grown man!" My mother, who was at home in Bowman, would know by morning. I could count on it. But this night, I reveled in freedom. When at about 10 or 11 o'clock the horn sounded again for promenading to stop, Sidney said "I'm staying at the preacher's tent. Where are you staying?" I answered that I was not staying at my relatives' tent, but had ridden out from Bowman with a cousin with whom I was expected to return. With my newly found abandon, I agreed to tell the cousin that I was riding the five miles to Bowman with Sidney. So away we went in his V-8 Ford out of the campground on the small sandy lane, past my grandparents' house and then on the moonlit dirt road between phalanxes of trees on either side. I sat primly against the car door on my side, but my heart was racing. Here I was with an older man who wanted to be with me just for me!

When we arrived at my house, he escorted me to the door, said a proper goodnight, and I went in to face the moment of truth. Needless to say, my mother was not pleased. She suspected Sidney of the most ulterior motives. When I asked whether I could accompany him the next day on his recruiting trip to see boys who lived on farms around Bowman, she said, "We'll see after I meet him." The next day she reluctantly agreed, but I had to be back before dark. That was easy, because Sidney had to drive back to Greenville that night. Mother's pronouncement after he left was, "I don't like him. He smiles too much. He seems insincere."

Sidney remained my only romantic interest throughout high

school. We exchanged a few cards during the next year, and in the summer I began to wait anxiously for him to return on a recruiting trip.

My family now lived on the main street of Bowman, and I watched for V-8 Fords, hoping he would be in each one. Finally, in late summer, Sidney came for a visit and we spent a chaste afternoon together, with me sitting in the car while he went into the farm houses to interview potential college candidates. Next, I saw him my senior year in high school when I went to a writing contest in Greenville, again, a short daytime tryst. I finally plucked up my nerve to invite him to escort me to my senior high school banquet, a grand affair at the hotel in Greenwood. One of my best friends lived at the hotel (her father was the manager), and the afternoon before the banquet we checked the register hourly to see whether he had arrived. Our excitement was at fever pitch. Lala had made me a beautiful white brocaded satin evening dress and she, unlike Mother, greeted Sidney warmly and we were off. I remember being a little concerned about appearing with an older man, but little else about the banquet. What I do remember was our ride around Greenwood after the banquet and his kiss on my forehead. I was transported for days!

I didn't see Sidney the next summer. By then he was at Duke Divinity School, and I was in summer school at the University of South Carolina. The next fall I caught a ride to Duke with friends going to a football game and spent a wonderful evening with him. We had no money so we just walked around the campus, listened outside the auditorium where one of the famous big bands was playing, went into the beautiful Duke Cathedral, and ended the evening by walking through a pine forest that must have been a part of the Duke Gardens. Anyway, it was here that Sidney put his arms around me and gave me my first real kiss. My college roommate had been coaching me on how to respond to a kiss. "Put your hands up around the back of the boy's head . . ." I forgot all the coaching; I just melted into his embrace. I was in love. At one in the morning I burrowed into the back seat with the car full of my friends, and we took the long trip back to Columbia. I didn't sleep a wink all the way back. I shut my eyes and relived the moment over and over, and for weeks I was walking around starry eyed.

During that year, Sidney and I exchanged a few letters and planned to meet at camp meeting (he was still recruiting students), but I couldn't go to Bowman that summer. There was a polio epidemic and Bowman was hit hard, even camp meeting was canceled. Somehow Sidney didn't get the message and drove the long trip to Bowman. When he missed me, I found out later, he went to see a young woman of his own age in St. George, a nearby town. I was furious with Mother for not letting me come home that summer. She kept telling me that the romance wasn't going anywhere, and if it did, I'd be bored to death being a preacher's wife in South Carolina. And furthermore, he smiled too much.

The next time I saw Sidney, I had finished medical school, was married and had a family. He was an army chaplain, had served in World War II, and had lived all over the world. Seven years ago, when I was 67 years old and he was almost eighty, I ran into him in Charleston. He was recently widowed and was grieving, but he was optimistic and still smiling. He and I drove to Bowman and took pictures of the campground, the tabernacle, and the choir where we met. It was a nostalgic trip, but we could both see that life had been good to us and that we had each made the right choices. Now, as I write this, it's July and camp meeting time and I'm wondering how Sidney is. Maybe I'll call him and hear his smiling voice.

* * * * * * * *

I finished high school on a Friday in June 1938 and entered the University of South Carolina, in Columbia, on the following Monday. This was not what I planned to do. I wanted to stay in Greenwood that summer and start college in the fall, but I didn't get to carry out my plans because of major changes in my family's situation. My brother Arthur Dow had moved to Columbia to work, and Mother decided to move to Columbia, where she managed to get a teaching job at a nearby orphanage. Daddy stayed in Bowman, living alone or, at times, with Catherine and Rhett. By this time, my father was deteriorating mentally and within the next few years had to be committed to the state mental hospital where he would live off and on for the rest of his life.

Before Mother could start her job, she had to take some refresher courses and insisted that I accompany her and start my college training immediately. There went my summer!

There were only two South Carolina schools that offered premedical courses to girls: Winthrop, a highly regimented, hard-working state school for girls, and the coeducational University of South Carolina that had the reputation of being very social. There was, of course, no possibility that my family could send me to an out-of-state school, so I opted for Winthrop; but Mother insisted that I go to the University. There were two probable reasons for her choice: she felt that I needed to be in a coeducational school, and since she was moving to Columbia to teach, she could keep an eye on me.

That first summer was dismal. The campus was full of teachers, but few students my own age. I had a dining room scholarship which kept me working behind a hot steam table in an unair-conditioned dining room. Even worse, I roomed with my mother. Rooming with one's mother is not exactly "going off to school," and I hated the whole setup.

Fortunately, the fall was better. I roomed in a house with seventeen other girls and began to feel like a college student. The University was on a beautiful old campus situated in the middle of Columbia. It was only a block from the impressive Capital building at the foot of Main Street. No one had or needed cars, so students walked everywhere. Columbia was a college town.

In 1938, the year I entered the University, the student body consisted of about 4,000 students, three-fourths men, one-fourth women. Its reputation of being a social school proved to be true. Fraternity and sorority activities were important. The boys were noted for being big drinkers and playing hard. I believe, however, that the majority of them had career goals and had some idea of how they would use their education, but the girls were different. Few of them planned to have careers. Those who planned to work were preparing to teach, be librarians, or do some type of clerical work. Nursing was a leading career choice in the 1930s and 40s, but girls preparing to go into nursing rarely went to the university. A few went to college for a year or two, but generally, they entered hospital-based nursing schools directly after finishing high school. Many of the girls I knew at the university planned to go back home and live with their parents until they got married. For them, the university was a kind of finishing school and a place to meet future husbands.

At first I was very disappointed to be in what I felt was such an uninspiring environment, but later I fit into the social life of the woman's dormitory and got my intellectual stimulation from being with the premedical students in class. I soon found that the professors were outstanding and the courses excellent. The premed curriculum was science-intense, but we were encouraged to take as many liberal arts courses as possible.

As much as I decried it, the university social life was probably good for me, and I began to be more like other girls. I let my short hair grow out, wore feminine clothes, learned to use slang, and to carry on light conversation. My roommate and dormitory mates proved to be wonderful friends, and we helped each other grow up. In the dormitory, we had talk sessions far into the night. The subject was generally sex and boys. Ironically, I was considered an expert on sex because my brother had given me a copy of *Sane Sex Life*, by Dr. Havelock Ellis, the Dr. Kinsey of the 1940s. I had devoured it from cover to cover, but I was still rather naive.

One night, the other girls shocked me by discussing "white slavery." I'd never heard of such a thing, but they assured me it was an ever present threat, because men abducted young women and forced them to be prostitutes. Every girl was supposed to know never to go to the movies alone and sit by a man. He might stab her with a drug-filled syringe and whisk her away never to be heard from again! In addition to supplying this valuable education, the other girls taught me to dance. I was not very well equipped in that area, since the Charleston was long out of style. My roommate had a bedside radio, and girls gathered in our room and waltzed, fox-trotted, tangoed, and jitterbugged to the music of the big bands: Glenn Miller, Artie Shaw, Sammy Kaye. We knew all the romantic lyrics of "Deep Purple," "Night and Day," "Stormy Weather."

It was an era of romance and sentimentality. Now, when I listen to these soft, sweet old songs, I think they are better than the loud, repetitious songs belted out today at thousands of decibels. And I remember innocent girls sitting around on dormitory beds singing, "Can't go on, everything I have is gone, stormy weather, me and my man ain't together . . . ;" "Night and day, you are the one, only you beneath the moon and under the sun . . . ;" and my special favorite, the steamy "Temptation," "You came, I was alone, I should have known, my heart was gone. You are temptation and I am yours."

After all of the dormitory coaching in the terpsichorean art, I joined Damas, the girls' dance club that existed for one purpose: to enable us to invite boys to two dances a year. This, in turn, led to reciprocal invitations to the boys' dances. During my years at the University, I dated a modest amount, but just with good friends and no romantic involvement. I was still daydreaming about Sidney. However, during my second year in summer school, I met another older man who would play a major role in my life.

I was taking all of organic chemistry in two hot, steamy sessions of summer school. Despite the high ceilings and big windows in the old chemistry building, the numerous Rube Goldberg arrangements of bunsen burners, retorts, and glass tubing made the laboratory a veritable sauna. The temperature and humidity were overwhelming. We spent five hours each day in this hot mist-filled environment, then went out into the 100° Columbia weather to study in our hot dormitory rooms.

Ten semester credits in organic chemistry in one summer was an unwise goal, and I retained little of what I learned that summer, but on one of those long hot mornings, a tall, handsome, mature looking man loomed up in the laboratory fog and introduced himself to me. He told me that his name was Joe Wyman, he was twenty-eight years old, and he was taking his last pre-med course so that he could go to medical school the coming fall. He later told me that he had been out of school working for a number of years and had only recently decided to go to medical school. He was from a family of doctors, but for some reason had resisted going to medical school at the usual age. Now, he was obviously concerned about his ability to be a student again.

At the time, I never knew why he was attracted to me. Later, when our relationship had become more casual, he said it was my legs; but I always suspected it was my intense preoccupation with being a doctor and my assumption that, of course, I could do it. Regardless of the reason, he invited me to go to a movie with him that night.

When I arrived back at the dormitory and announced that I was going out with an older man (I was then seventeen) there was a great ferment. The other girls insisted that I not wear saddle shoes and socks – it had to be heels and stockings. They were also adamant that they apply my makeup and dictated that under no circumstances was I to wear my glasses. That evening, my "ladies in waiting" applied my makeup, supervised my dressing, and confiscated my glasses.

At seven o'clock, I was paged for a visitor in the lobby. Trembling, I stumbled my way down the stairs and peered across what to me was a dim room (I was so near sighted, I could hardly see the furniture much less recognize a person). I walked across the lobby, hands outstretched to welcome Joe with what I thought was a gracious adult gesture. Suddenly, my brother's voice boomed out, ""For goodness sakes, Martha, what is the matter with you? I've brought your laundry to you." Thoroughly abashed, I stomped back up the stairs and retrieved my glasses, leaving on the makeup and high heels. When the second call came I went down, hands by my sides, to meet Joe. Fortunately, the glasses didn't do me in, because that was the first of many good times Joe and I would have together in the future.

During college I was growing up socially and learning to be like other girls, but throughout that time, my driving force was my goal to attend medical school; nothing was going to get in my way. I also felt the necessity for finishing the premed curriculum as quickly as possible because my brother was financing my college years and it was costing him $250 per semester, including tuition, room, board, and books. Although this figure seems paltry by today's standards, it was a healthy sum in the late 1930s when he was making about $200 a month. I took the maximum number of courses per semesters and went to summer school for three years.

In the fall of 1939, those of us in premed who would have the requisite semester hours began to discuss applying to medical school. Today, it is not unusual for students to apply to as many as four or five schools but, in our class, few people applied anywhere but the Medical College of South Carolina. Times were still hard and most of us were concerned about raising enough money to go even to our state school. Not only that, we wanted to go to Charleston, to our own medical school where primary emphasis was training doctors to practice in South Carolina. I doubt whether any of us ever thought we would practice anywhere else.

In any event, we took the medical school entrance examination. It was long, but not terribly hard, and surprisingly light in the sciences; it was geared to vocabulary, comprehension and retentiveness instead. In addition to the examination, we were required to write an essay on why we wanted to be a doctor, a subject that always made me defensive. I don't remember what I wrote, but I must have said something right, because early in the winter of 1940, I received an invitation for an interview. So on a Saturday I borrowed mother's car and drove the 120 miles to Charleston. I parked outside the old brick building, then the only building at the medical college, and across the street from Roper Hospital, an old broken down charity hospital. I walked up two or three worn steps into a broad hall and then a short distance to a dark wooden door with a name above it – Cyril P. O'Driscoll. I knocked and was admitted by Dr. O'Driscoll into a cluttered, book-filled room smelling of pipe tobacco. Dr. O'Driscoll wore a long speckled tan lab coat over his seventy-year-old body. He had a big rugged face, piercing eyes, his teeth were yellowed from the pipe clenched between them. A thin line of spittle ran out of the corner of his mouth. He ordered me to, "Sit down, young lady."

I don't remember very much about the interview, except that I realized that this man had total control over whether or not I would be admitted. There was no admissions committee and he had no formal title, such as, dean of admissions. Today, all medical schools have admission committees on which as many as fifty faculty members spend countless hours, including many weekends, reviewing applications and interviewing candidates. For us, there was just Cyril P. O'Driscoll, Professor of Anatomy for about forty years, the person who selected students. In spite of my fear, still vividly palpable over fifty years later, three details of that interview stand out: two were statements he made, and the third was a question he didn't ask.

His two comments were: "You have a strong letter of recommendation from Charlie Mercer (Professor of Physics at the University), and students who Charlie Mercer recommends always do well;" and "You're too young to go to medical school (I was eighteen), but you're good in English and Latin so I may take you." He didn't ask the inevitable question of that era: "Why should I waste a place on a woman when you probably won't ever work anyway?" He didn't have that prejudice. I seem to remember that there was a quota for women and for Jewish students and a definite quota for out-of-state students. Of course, the question of black students never arose. They went to schools for blacks, such as Howard University in Washington.

After my nerve-wracking interview, I called Joe Wyman and was aghast to hear that he was studying on Saturday. I didn't stay for Saturday night (I found out later that Saturday night was a very different matter) and instead drove back to Columbia.

After posting our essays and getting through our interviews, my colleagues and I, back at the University, waited to hear about our acceptance or rejection. One beautiful spring day, the rumor spread across the campus that the notices had arrived in our mail boxes. I rushed over to the University post office and opened my box to pull out a smudged penny postcard that said, "You have been accepted by the Medical College of South Carolina. Please report to the registrar on September 16, 1940."

And then a terrible calamity occurred. I failed trigonometry! I couldn't believe it. When I looked at the list of successful "passers" on the bulletin board, my name was missing. In a state of shock, I went into the professor's office and, with the arrogance of youth said, "There's been a mistake. My name has been left off the list." His reply was, "There's no mistake, young lady. You failed." Crestfallen and horrified, I limped back to the dormitory. What was I going to do? I had to have those three credits to go to medical school. And in a panic, as I reviewed the situation, I realized that it was, of course, all my fault. I hated math and had simply not studied. Somehow I had to learn a lot in a hurry and try to get the professor to permit me to take a re-exam.

First, I went to see the professor again and abjectly pled for a re-exam. After a long period of silence, he agreed to give me another chance a week hence. That gave me seven days to learn a semester's trigonometry. My brother, an engineer and a whiz at math, came over each evening that week and tutored me. On a Saturday morning, I sweated through the re-exam, and on Monday learned that I had passed, just barely, but I got those three credits. Over fifty years later, I have nightmares about taking a math exam, knowing absolutely nothing, and failing.

Now came the search for money to go to medical school. I still had to go to summer school for the third summer to complete my 90 semester hours, so there was no way to earn any money during the summer. Nationwide, there were very few scholarships, and most of them were for men, and there were none for men or women at the Medical College of South Carolina. I investigated every possibility, and it became apparent I would have to borrow money from some individual. My mother and I, together and separately, went to a number of businessmen and pillars of the community in Orangeburg and Greenwood. Nobody wanted to take a chance on a long shot like a girl going to medical school. Would she pass? Would she really work in medicine? Would she repay the loan?

August came and I still had no money. Finally, in desperation, my mother and I went to see Dr. Jane Bruce Guignard, one of the first women doctors in South Carolina. She was then in her seventies. Although she was from a prominent Columbia family, it was necessary for her to teach school for a number of years to earn the money for her education at Women's Medical College in Philadelphia. She was very familiar with the difficulty of financing a medical education for a woman, but she was tough (she had to be to have become one of the most respected physicians in Columbia). She interviewed me rigorously and it was evident that she didn't like my mother and thought I might be a fly-by-night dilettante. She suggested that I go to the University for another year and then go to Woman's Medical or Johns Hopkins. She asked me how I felt about working as a teacher or medical technician and saving the money to go to medical school. I answered that I thought it was more logical to borrow money, get my M.D. degree, and pay the money back. After an intense, grueling interview, she said, "If you can get the money for the first year and pass, I'll lend you the money for the last three years."

Now I come to the part of this story that amazes me each time I think of it. Although a lot of people believed in me, someone in my life did so to an extraordinary and unselfish degree.

It was Lala who came through with a generous offer: "I'll mortgage my home to lend you the money for the first year." That doesn't sound as generous and daring in 1994 as it did in 1940. Today, everybody has a mortgage, but having a mortgage in the 1930s and early 1940s was a frightening thing. Owning your home outright was very important. People who owned their homes during the depression had a much better chance of surviving the financial crises than those who didn't. I remember a statement that was almost a litany: "They had a mortgage on their home, so they lost it." For my aunt to mortgage her only possession, and to bet on an eighteen-year-old girl to make good and repay the mortgage was a brave, loving thing to do. Lots of people believed in me, but Lala really believed in me! Many times when medical school got very tough and the work load seemed insurmountable, or when I was tempted to play too much, I thought I can't let my family down and I can't let Lala down.

Chapter 3

Medical School at Last

THE MOST FREQUENT QUESTION asked of a young person aspiring to be a doctor is, "Why do you want to be a doctor?" It's a hard question generally requiring a complex answer, more complex than most inquirers really want to hear, but I've been asked it by so many young career women that I have endeavored here to analyze it for myself. I realize that there were at least four influences that had convinced me that I wanted to be a doctor: my interest in biology, the maternal approval I received for this ambition, the health problems I recognized during my growing up in Bowman, and my observations of the life of our country physician, Dr. Black.

My innate interest in biology, especially microbiology, and my strong desire for discovering new things, made me an avid reader of scientific books and articles about microbes and their discoverers. Reading *Arrowsmith* and *Microbe Hunters* when I was in high school had made a lasting impression on me. I wanted to discover new things about microorganisms and the way they produced disease.

This questing attitude was encouraged by my family, especially my mother. Mother loved the idea that I wanted to be a doctor and reinforced the belief that it would be possible. There is no doubt that a part of my intense, single-minded determination to be a doctor was augmented by her approval and encouragement. Also, the interest and admiration that my wanting to be a doctor inspired in other adults was a social crutch for me, compensating in some measure for my feeling of inadequacy in peer relationships. My desire to be a doctor was my claim to fame.

Unquestionably, the large amount of illness that I observed while I was growing up made me aware of the need for good medical care. One group of experiences left an indelible impression on me. In 1935, when I was thirteen and still living in Bowman with my parents (before moving to Greenwood with Aunt Lala), Mother had a government-sponsored job as a part of a survey of the health needs in Orangeburg County, and often I accompanied her on her survey trips. It was the first time I had seen the effects of dire poverty. I'd heard about people losing their farms because they couldn't make the mortgage payments or couldn't buy seed or fertilizer, but I hadn't seen the way many people had to live in broken down, unpainted shacks, children running around the yard half naked and shoeless even in winter. The medical problems were appalling. We saw seriously ill people, blind people, crippled people and emaciated children covered with crusting and weeping sores. Many of them had never been to a doctor. I learned that these people were not simply "shiftless," as popular opinion would have me believe. Their plights were due to no jobs, no money, no transportation, and most importantly, no education. I learned early of the crucial relationship between health care and social conditions. I also learned that preventive medical care was far down the list of priorities for the really poor. Care came after the necessities for survival – food, shelter, and clothing. Observing all this misery convinced me that someday I wanted to do something about the health problems of the poor.

I would like to say that nurture and the desire to help people was the main impetus to my wanting to be a doctor, but I don't think I truly understood the significance of my exposure to the harsher realities of being poor in the south until later. However, I did know that I wanted to do something of value for the community in which I lived and to earn its respect.

Many medical school applicants related that they were influenced by relatives who were doctors or by respected physicians in their hometowns. My only physician relative was a great uncle who was killed in the Civil War, and I know very little about him. However, I believe that I was influenced by our Bowman family physician, Dr. Black. My most vivid memories of him are house calls he made when I was sick. He had a gruff bedside manner. Pulling up a chair next to my bed, he would question Mother about my symptoms. Then he gave me a thorough physical, reached into his stiff black bag, produced some terrible tasting medicine and wrote a prescription in Latin. He charged Mother two dollars for these visits, with the comment, "Pay me when you can."

Occasionally, Mother would take me to his office for a blood test. His office was downstairs in a brick building that opened directly on to the sandy sidewalk of Main Street. He and his family lived upstairs over the office. If the card hanging in the window said "Doctor In," we'd ring the bell and were admitted into his bare, white, scrupulously clean office. I was mesmerized by the room where I imagined Dr. Black treated all sorts of ills – stab wounds, snake bites, arms hanging from a farm accident. I watched him examine my blood under the microscope, wishing I could look through that wonderful instrument.

Dr. Black had no scheduled office hours, and I doubt whether anyone ever made an appointment with him. Most of the time, he was out making house calls in the town or throughout the countryside around Bowman. If his card said "Doctor Out," and it was necessary to leave a message, one walked up the wooden steps on the outside of the building and rang the bell for Mrs. Black. She always seemed to be at home and always answered, "I'll tell the Doctor."

When I became close friends with Dr. Black's daughter, Anna Lou, I got to accompany them on his house calls out in the country. Anna Lou and I went along mostly because we wanted to ride in the rumble seat of his Model A Ford. Of course, I didn't see the patients, but I observed how he was paid for his services. When anxious family members, accompanying Dr. Black out to the car, explained that they couldn't pay for the visit, he would cast his eye across the garden and the barnyard and the bill would then be settled by his receiving some chickens, a ham, maybe a bushel of peaches.

Today, I am amazed at what Dr. Black was able to accomplish, given the fact that he had no nurse, no secretary, no laboratory, and no hospital in which to work. He had his eyes, his ears, a black bag containing a stethoscope, a blood pressure cuff, and an instrument for examining eyes and ears, and assorted medicines (such as digitalis, adrenalin and cough syrups). In his office he had a few surgical instruments, material for plaster casts, a fluoroscope, a sterilizer, and a microscope for looking at blood cells and urine. Many people in Bowman thought of Dr. Black as being cold and remote; they didn't acknowledge that he was also available day or night, unless he was out on a call. I truly doubt whether the man took off a day in his life.

As I think about Dr. Black, I realize that for all his hard work and long hours, the way he and his family lived appealed to me. At ten years old, I was very aware that Anna Lou had nice clothes, took music lessons, and ate well even during the depression – chicken, pork, beef, and fresh vegetables were often served. Each morning, their doorstep was graced with five quarts of milk for their family of five, while at our house we had one quart for the five of us. To my ten-year-old mind, the connection between an ample table and a closet full of nice clothes had to do with having a skill that was always needed. I was keenly aware of the tenuous nature of my parents' skills – farming and teaching – and I became determined to earn the sense of financial freedom I saw represented by Dr. Black and his family. Also, I wanted to be a respected member of the community.

* * * * * * * *

A Saturday in 1940 began what would prove to be some of the happiest years of my life. I was eighteen years old and was truly leaving home for the first time in my life because, although I had not lived at home during my high school and college years, my mother had maintained a tight control over me. Now I would be a hundred and twenty miles from that control.

Joe Wyman, a medical school friend of his, and I took off for Charleston as Mother waved, exhorting Joe, "Take care of her for me." We rode through the sand hills, the red hills, across the flat coastal low country, and then along the beautiful River Road with ancient moss-hung oaks arching across it. There we met the harbinger of Charleston – the plough mud smell of the marshes. Spread before us were the green of the grasses, the blue of the wide Ashley River, and the shining white of the bridge leading into the city. At that moment, I fell in love with Charleston – a love I still have. Half jokingly, I say that if I'm good, when I die God will let me go to Charleston, with its tidal rivers and marshes, in lieu of heaven, with its angels and harps.

My escorts took me by the medical college to register and then to 96 Bull Street, the home of the Ravenel sisters, the traditional place for women medical students to live. Ninety-six Bull Street was a classical Charleston "single house." It was a three-story house only one room wide, but many rooms deep. The entrance was directly on the sidewalk with no front yard, a startling difference from most Southern homes.

Here there was a door with a bell. This door opened onto a high flight of stairs leading to a broad piazza that overlooked a side garden. Off of the piazza was the real door of the house. Joe rang the downstairs bell, took my bag up the steps, rang the upstairs bell, and introduced me to Miss Florence Ravenel. Miss Florence showed me into the second floor which I later learned was often the main living area of Charleston houses. Here there was a stiffly formal living room, a big formal dining room, and the bedroom that I was to share with another medical student. The kitchen must have been on that floor, too, but as far as I can remember, I never saw it. Our style of living was far too formal to permit that. At the Ravenel's we were always "guests," never boarders, and all of the time I lived there I was always "Miss Dukes," not Martha.

Miss Florence explained that I would be rooming with Miss Kathleen Riley, a senior medical student. Then she left me to settle into a large high-ceilinged, airy room with big windows overlooking the neighbor's fragrant garden. The room seemed all white – white walls, white gauzy curtains, two white iron beds, and white bedspreads. It contained one small desk, a desk chair, and an easy chair. Opposite the windows there was an enormous mahogany armoire, and in the middle of the room was a pot-bellied stove. Off the pristine white bedroom was an equally pristine white bathroom with a footed tub. There were meager arrangements for study, but this was a wonderful suite and I loved it.

Promptly at six, a bell announced supper which proved to be an interesting experience and a preview of future meals at 96 Bull Street. Miss Florence settled quietly into her place at the foot of the table and Miss Isobel, the other Ravenel sister, presided at the head of the table. She was formidable, her hair piled severely on the top of her head, pince-nez glasses resting on her nose with the chain pinned to her rigidly corseted ample bosom. She was the epitome of a D.A.R. president. Miss Nina (Neen) Ravenel, the ninety-year-old aunt, fluttered to her chair and lit between the "guests" like a tiny, frail, hyperactive bird. Miss Isobel said the blessing, the maid passed the food, and the conversation proceeded decorously between the other two guests, a senior medical student and a graduate student, until Miss Neen offered to take me, the newcomer, on an outing. "Miss Dukes, after supper how would you like to go for a ride around the battery in my machine?"

This apparently innocent offer caused obvious distress to the sisters. The machine was an ancient Model T Ford which Miss Neen drove with much noise and great abandon. Miss Isobel and Miss Florence were terribly upset by their aunt's insistence on making a "spectacle of herself." Soon, I came to know that Miss Neen's greatest joy was their discomfiture. I learned, also, that when meals became too staid and quiet, we students could count on Miss Neen to say something outrageous to scandalize her nieces. We enjoyed her company, but on this first night I asked Miss Neen for a rain check, because I had other plans.

About eight o'clock, Joe came by to introduce me to the social side of medical school. As he had promised my mother, he was taking care of me. We walked across the piazza, down the flight of stairs and through the street door into the misty night. The soft seductive air was filled with rattling of palmetto fronds, and the gnarled oak trees cast deep shadows on the lantern-lit sidewalks as we walked the short block to the AKK house where the fraternity was having an opening-of-the-year party. The house was a splendid antebellum mansion set in a beautiful garden. Curved steps with a handsome wrought iron railing led up to a broad veranda washed by light coming through the open door and floor length French windows. Here couples were courting and small groups of people were talking and drinking. We entered a spacious hall with a splendid staircase winding up to the second and third floors from which sounds of revelry floated down. Here, Joe paused to advise me that nice girls didn't go upstairs in the fraternity house. Conviviality reigned in the dining room, and there was music and dancing in the living room. Joe introduced me to a few people and then left me to socialize on my own, no problem in that group.

There were many Charleston girls and girls visiting from various parts of the state to share this last carefree weekend with their men friends, but still there was an excess of men – a great situation! We waltzed, we tangoed, we jitter bugged to the strains of "Blue Moon," "In The Mood," "Sentimental Journey," and sometimes we just sat and watched as the least inhibited people performed exhibition numbers. A sophomore student gave a fantastic rendition of "rubber legs," a form of jitter bugging that few people ever mastered. The music went on and on. More and more purple passion (grape juice and grain alcohol) was consumed. I didn't drink alcohol in those days, but I was intoxicated by the atmosphere of gay abandon. At some time during the evening, a tall, gangly boy came up to me and said, "I'm Tucker Weston. Will you go downtown with me tomorrow?" When I hesitated, he added, "I have a car!" I don't remember the end of the evening or walking back to 96 Bull Street. I probably floated. It was a magic time in a magic place!

The next day, Tucker arrived in his Model A Ford, already a collector's item, which he made backfire to announce his arrival as if anyone could miss the rattle of that car's approach! He showed me downtown Charleston, the beautiful old historic district situated on a peninsula between two great tidal rivers (the Ashley and the Cooper), and the austere Citadel where he had gone to college. Thus, began a short innocent romance that lasted only a few months, but began a friendship that has lasted a lifetime. We were instantly infatuated with each other and I was very relieved that I was able to care about a person my own age. I had begun to fear that I had a father fixation and could be attracted only to older men. Tucker and I had a wonderful, uncomplicated romance that just gradually dwindled away. Neither of us felt deserted or bad. Thinking back, I suppose that Tucker met the girl he subsequently married, and I became more involved with other men. All in all, it was a perfect first love affair – all joy and no pain. Tucker is now an orthopedist in Columbia and very active in the medical affairs of South Carolina, but in those days he was just a big, wholesome, happy young man.

On Sunday night, the night after the memorable fraternity party, my roommate arrived. She was a short, somewhat plump, pretty girl who fit her Irish name, Kathleen Riley. It took me only a few minutes to recognize the vast gulf that lay between being a senior medical student and being a freshman. Not only was there the gulf of medical experience, but Kathleen was six years older than I and more sophisticated and mature. My first impression was that she was a real egghead, and she thought I was a playgirl. Both impressions were wrong. We soon learned that each of us was deadly serious and idealistic about being a doctor and both of us loved to have a good time. In the next few weeks, we discovered that we enjoyed the same literature and the same music and shared a similar sense of humor. On that first evening, Kathleen became my role model by quickly explaining that as women, we had to work hard in medicine, harder than the men for equal recognition, and we both agreed that we were determined to avoid being stereotyped as the typical woman doctor. At that time, the common concept of a woman doctor was a female with short hair, little or no make up, dressed in a severely man-tailored suit and bulky low-heeled oxfords. We were bent on dressing well and conducting ourselves in a feminine manner to do our part in dispelling this image.

On Monday morning, Kathleen left resplendent in a short starched white coat, stethoscope protruding from the pocket at just the right angle. I dressed carefully in a pretty suit, low-heeled pumps and stockings. Gone were the dirty saddle shoes and the bobby socks of college days. Billy McCaw, a friend from premed days at the University, came to walk the few blocks to the medical college with me. He was a freshman and as awed as I; and he, too, was dressed according to the unspoken dress code – coat, tie, polished shoes. We walked along the wide Ashley River and entered the auditorium at one end of the school.

The faculty was assembled with the dean (one dean, no president, no young men in grey flannel suits representing administration). The dean was white haired, erect, and distinguished in a gleaming white suit. The one hundred sixty members of the student body listened to a brief, dignified welcome and then we went to our classes. The 46 members of the freshman class, 44 men and two women, met in a small intimate classroom presided over by Cyril P. O'Driscoll. Here we heard how it was really going to be! He told us in no uncertain terms that we were now in a professional school; we were privileged to be there and we had one chance to pass all subjects our freshman year or we were out. He delivered this message to us in a booming voice and the small intimate room became too intimate and seemed dangerous. Each of us was given a bag of bones. It looked like a flour sack and rattled when we walked. We were to live with this bag of bones for the next two weeks and were to bring it back and forth to class each day. We also were issued a skull to keep at home. I kept mine on the bureau in our bedroom, much to the horror of the black maid. Each day when she was cleaning, she covered it with a white towel, presumably to ward off the "evil eye."

We had no courses but osteology (the study of bones) for the first two weeks, and we had one mentor, Cyril P. O'Driscoll. We lived with him, the bones, and *Cunningham's Anatomy*, a tome of alarming size. He assured us that we would know every bump and notch on all 204 bones in the human body, and before the year was over, we would read all 1,332 pages of the anatomy book – not once, but many times – and would commit many of them to memory. Also he told us that during the next four years we would acquire a new vocabulary of thousands of words. And all of this was true. Each day, we came into the room fearing that this would be the day we would be called on to recite. Dr. O'Driscoll, spittle running down his chin, would bellow out a name and throw a bone to an unlucky student: "Describe this bone." And if the victim hesitated over the new words so foreign to our tongues, he would yell, "Man, bet your money and sleep in the street!" or "Shoot, Luke or give up the gun!" None of us thought that we would ever become facile in terms such as antero-lateral or postero-lateral. I've often wondered why we needed the minute detail we were required to learn in those first two weeks, but I think the course must have been designed to teach us discipline.

Looking back, those two weeks of osteology were a hardening process, a testing of one's mettle or maybe a baptism by fire. At the end of the two weeks, we took our first exam – one of the eighteen oral anatomy exams we would have in the first year. After this first exam, we were taken to the big dissecting room and given our cadavers lying on the rows of dissecting tables. This was the moment we had dreaded most. We weren't sure we could touch these cold, dead bodies; but we did and at that moment the smell of formaldehyde entered our sinuses, permeated our lab coats (we now wore hideous, long, tan, speckled lab coats over our still careful dress), and seemed to penetrate our skin. For the next nine months when we raised our forks to our mouths, we would smell formaldehyde on our hands. No soap was strong enough or perfumed enough to remove it. During those first few months, most of us had trouble eating.

We dissected and studied all morning, every morning, and we formed lifelong bonds with our dissecting partners. My partner, Dr. Williams McIver (Billy) Bryan, and I have an affection that bridges years and distances. Billy Bryan and I spent long hours together during weekday classes, on Saturdays, Sundays, and sometimes at night. It was not possible to complete our work during regular hours and often, there were many teams in the dissecting room with us. The doors were never locked and the lights were never turned off. Billy and I dissected and we talked over our cadaver. The remarks were mostly things like, "Dukes, do you have a branch of the artery on your side like this one on my side?" or "Billy, what in the world is this nerve doing here?" But Billy found time to explain to me many things about the art of courtship. He was a wonderful teacher. He was suave and accomplished in that area and, most important, he really liked women. He gave me assurance about my own social abilities.

No description of the gross anatomy course would be complete without a description of the oral exams. Every two weeks we were assigned dissection of a certain part of the body, and at the end of that time, we were grilled by either Dr. O'Driscoll of the biting tongue, or by the chairman of the department, Dr.

Arthur Lassek, an austere and forbidding man. It was hard to decide who was worse, but I believe most of us preferred Dr. O'Driscoll's sarcasm to Dr. Lassek's frigid manner. Dr. O'Driscoll would walk up to the table, point with his scalpel and say, "Mr. Bryan, describe the descending aorta," or "Miss Dukes, tell me about the mitral valve." One's partner listened intently, knowing he would be called on to agree or disagree and knowing his time was coming. The stress of these experiences was so great that one of our classmates vomited before each session, and another cried on several occasions. After a few months, one of our classmates dropped out and joined the air force. We always believed it was because he thought that combat would be less stressful than the oral anatomy exams. The rest of us plodded on to pass our freshman year.

In spite of the hard work and stress, I was very happy because I knew I was in the right place. I really enjoyed the work and was feeling good about myself. Here I felt accepted and no longer different from my peers. I was just one of the freshman class. We were in the trenches together, working like crazy, but laughing about the eccentricities of our professors and our difficulties. Medical students have to laugh. It's necessary for survival.

Chapter 4

Surviving Medical School

WHEN I WROTE THAT my years in medical school were a happy time, I must have conveniently forgotten my sophomore year. It was deadly – nine more months of basic science travail – physiology, pharmacology, biochemistry, microbiology, and pathology! Some of these courses could have been fascinating. Certainly physiology was when we read the text and learned how the human body functioned and the marvelous interactions of the organ systems. But three of our professors were septuagenarians, and we felt that their information was at least twenty years out of date, so we had to memorize their obsolete notes in order to pass, while trying to glean contemporary information from the texts. This difficult task was compounded by our constant fear of failing. Failing one course meant taking the entire year over. My memories of this difficult period are refreshed by a quotation from a recently published history of the Medical University of South Carolina which vividly describes the situation.

> The first 50 years of the 20th century were years of confrontation between the faculty and the medical students. Students lived in perpetual fear of flunking. No student was certain of graduation until his name was read out by the dean at

> a convocation at the end of the school year. When a student flunked, he or she stayed flunked. There was no due process . . . The four years of medical school were in part a siege of controlled terror (Worthington et al. 1991).

As students, we survived this reign of terror because we were suffering together. We commiserated with each other, complained bitterly, plotted terrible things we would like to do to the professors, and laughed.

Our only redeeming course was pathology taught by Dr. Kenneth Lynch, the first person to link asbestosis to lung cancer. Pathology can be dull and a mere litany of diseases as they appear at the autopsy table, but Dr. Lynch excelled in his knowledge of the pathogenesis of disease (the mechanisms by which damage occurs, and the body's responses to noxious agents and events). I hesitate to say that Dr. Lynch made the subject "come alive," but his clear, inspiring teaching influenced my approach to diagnosis and management throughout my career.

A separate course, clinical pathology was devoted to laboratory diagnosis. It was very thorough and lasted a full year. The professor was extremely demanding, and a passing grade was hard won. We examined blood, urine, stool, and gastric juice. Countless hours were spent studying amoebae and other intestinal parasites, and every student had to master the art of diagnosing the three major types of malaria. We performed serology for typhoid, typhus, and brucellosis. Clinical pathology was tedious and we hated it, but when we entered our junior year and began working with patients, we knew which tests were appropriate and how to interpret the results. Today, much less emphasis is placed on teaching laboratory diagnosis, and frequently students arrive at the bedside sadly lacking in such fundamental information. Often they know more about expensive CAT scans than about ordinary blood tests. Many times on teaching rounds I have wished that my students had been required to have more solid grounding in laboratory diagnosis before beginning their clinical training. Fifty years later I appreciate the intensive introduction to laboratory tests, but at the time, clinical pathology was just one more burdensome course.

During our second year in medical school, our interest in

studying was flagging. We were tired of learning basic science and of acquiring the tools of the trade, and longed to begin dealing with patients. Today, students are introduced to clinical medicine much earlier than they were fifty years ago, sometimes seeing patients during the latter part of the first year or early in the second. But in our second year, the only introduction to patient care was a short course in physical diagnosis where the importance of history taking was stressed and where we learned the elements of physical examination by examining each other. The two girls were lucky to have each other to examine, but needless to say, we got lots of offers from the boys.

Not only was this second year tough for me academically, it was also tough emotionally. Billy McCaw and I were fast friends, and I was still spending time with my friend, Joe, but in the late fall his old girl friend had reentered the picture. I gave her as much competition as possible, but to my great sorrow, she and Joe were married in January. I was heartbroken and "carried the torch" for him for a long time. That was my last serious romantic involvement during medical school.

Suddenly, at midpoint of the sophomore year, the tedium of our lives was interrupted by something vastly more important. On Sunday, December 7, 1941, I was in my room studying when the shocking news about the attack on Pearl Harbor was announced on the radio. Immediately, the urgent need for medical personnel changed medical schools and hospitals. Primarily, it changed the schedules of medical students and house officers (interns and residents). The content of training did not change; it was merely compressed into shorter periods. Medical schools adopted a year-round program so that students could be graduated in three years rather than four. Ours was a transitional class. We had only one summer off and would graduate in three and a half years.

One welcome change for the male medical students was an improvement in their financial situation. They were inducted in the army as privates first class, or in the navy as midshipmen and they were allowed to finish medical school receiving tuition, books, uniforms, and a living allowance. In the early forties, most of the students at the Medical College of South Carolina were on very tight budgets. Many worked at part-time jobs in order to stay in school. Some were night shift orderlies, some night watchmen, and four of my classmates were guards on the Cooper River bridge. Going to school and working was extremely difficult, so the financial support from the service was a great boon. But it never occurred to the women that we should have the same opportunity. There were nurses in the armed services, but no women doctors. The WACS (Women's Army Corps) and the WAVES (Women Accepted for Volunteer Emergency Service) didn't come into existence until late in our medical school years and even then women's medical education was not subsidized. Clearly the government policy was a case of sex discrimination, but at the time I did not recognize it as such. It never occurred to me. I just realized that I would not have to go overseas with combat troops. It was taken for granted that men went to battle and women kept the home fires burning.

Charleston was greatly changed by the war. It changed from a quiet Southern city to a busy war time seaport. The navy yard went into round-the-clock production, the harbor bustled with ships going in and out, and the usually empty streets were full of sailors and soldiers. Buckets of sand were put on rooftops in case of fire, black out curtains hung at the windows, and walking on the beaches after sundown was prohibited and enforced by military police on horseback. Rationing went into effect with coupons for gasoline, shoes, sugar, meat, butter, and other things, but nobody complained. The atmosphere was one of intense patriotism, the most amazing aspect of which was the maintenance of secrecy. Signs were posted everywhere carrying warnings like, "Loose Lips Sink Ships." From time to time, wounded foreign sailors were admitted to the city's hospital, but we were not permitted to ask them questions. We just helped take care of them. Somehow, we knew that one group of sailors was from a Portuguese tanker, but it was not until after the war that we learned that German submarines had been captured or sunk in the coastal waters just off of Charleston. I often wonder whether today, in this era of rapid communication and the insistence of the news media that everybody is entitled to know everything instantly, the United States could ever achieve such remarkable silence.

At the beginning of my junior year, I was twenty and began

to rebel against the restrictions and formality of life at the Ravenel's house. Despite my mother's and Dr. Guignard's displeasure, I decided with my roommate, Ann Harper, to move elsewhere. Through Billy McCaw, we learned that Dr. Barney Baker, one of the three Doctors Baker who owned Baker Memorial Hospital, was looking for someone to live in his Charleston house while his family moved to their beach house for the summer. We rushed over to the hospital and struck an instant deal. Now we had a lovely house with no chaperon and a living room and garden for entertaining.

It was a grand summer and entertain, we did. Ann had a thing about men in navy uniforms and was especially enamored of ensigns and lieutenant J.G.s. I don't remember how we met them, but there was a parade of them through our sumptuous establishment. Ann also became very familiar with the Carolina Yacht Club where naval officers had guest privileges.

All of this was very innocent, since neither Ann nor I could entertain any idea of marriage, although many of our college friends were now getting married. In fact, there was a rash of marriages among the male medical students, because soon the men would be going overseas and there was a sense of urgency. But Ann had to complete her course in medical technology and I had to finish medical school. I knew that if Dr. Guignard got the slightest hint of my having any serious romantic involvement, she would cut me off without a sou! I wanted to get married someday, but I was resolved to finish school and my residency training before considering marriage, another five or six years hence.

Our class was now in the clinical years, dealing with patients, but contrary to the custom today, we had concentrated didactic lectures. These lasted from eight in the morning until one in the afternoon – obstetrics and gynecology, general surgery, internal medicine, pediatrics, and psychiatry. The majority of the lectures were very good. Many of our teachers were practicing physicians who volunteered their time, and their lectures were organized and practical. Our only real problem was heat rash on our seats from the long hours of sitting in hot unair-conditioned rooms never designed for use in the Charleston summer. We had an afternoon break from 1:00 to 3:00 P.M., in keeping with the southern custom of having a big dinner at midday and a nap until 3:00. At 3:00, we went to clinics where we saw patients until 7:00 P.M. At night and on weekends, we were on call in rotation for patients. Many medical schools in the 1990s do not call students after 6:00 or 7:00 in the evening in order to give them time to study, but there was no such concern for students at the Medical College of South Carolina in the 1940s. We were there to learn to be doctors and doctors had to learn to work at night and to do without sleep!

In September the Bakers returned home, and Ann and I went our separate ways – Ann to live with some other girls, and I to room alone where I could get more studying done. My days of frenetic social life were over, and now, studying was a pleasure because most of it was providing information needed for understanding patient problems.

In most respects, the clinical years in medical school in the 1940s were similar to those in the 1990s. We learned primarily by working with patients under strict supervision. The medical student was the lowest member of a team that consisted of one or more house officers (interns or residents) and the attending physician. The medical student's assignment was to obtain a complete history and to perform a thorough physical examination. At Roper Hospital, our teaching hospital, obtaining a complete history was often a difficult task. All of our patients were indigent, many were vague or confused about their medical histories, and to compound the problem, many of them spoke Gullah, the dialect of African-Americans who lived on the sea islands of South Carolina. Gullah has a glossary of only about five hundred words, some African, some Elizabethan English, and some just lazily spoken English in the common vernacular. There seems to be no neuter gender, all objects being referred to as he or she or just "e." Not only does Gullah contain unique words, it is also spoken rapidly in an unusual cadence. Today the dialect has been diluted by increased communication and the advent of bridges and causeways, so that it is easier to understand. But in my days in medical school, it was still necessary to master at least the rudiments of Gullah in order to take a good history and to work with these patients from the islands. One day I was questioning an elderly black man when he said, "Doc,

I gonna cascade." When I didn't respond promptly, he repeated the statement more urgently, "I gonna cascade!" Not knowing what he meant, I replied, "Well, go ahead and cascade." With that he grabbed the basin on the bedside table and vomited copiously. When I consulted Webster's dictionary, I found the second definition of cascade to be "to vomit (rare colloq.)." I had the advantage of having learned some Gullah from my father's stories, and by my senior year I spoke it fluently, a great help in my work.

In addition to the language barrier, another difficulty we had in history taking was our self consciousness. Many ears listened to our fumbling questions, since all our patients were in big open wards. If necessary, curtains could be pulled around individual beds for visual privacy, but there was no auditory privacy. When the patient we were questioning was slow in responding, the patient in the next bed, who had his hand cupped behind his ear to hear better, might volunteer an answer or offer an opinion. The old timers in the ward were well aware of our inexperience, and to our chagrin, enjoyed giving the medical students as much help as possible.

Frequently, the patients we were examining assisted us as well. We were terribly anxious, because we were both inept and under pressure to be extremely thorough. Woe be to the student who missed a murmur or a small skin blemish that might be "a minor medical pearl," indicating some serious underlying problem. Here the patients were very helpful by giving us unsolicited information about what the house officers had found. In our inexperienced hands, the history and physical and the entry on the chart took up to two hours, and then we were off to the lab bench to perform a blood count, urinalysis, sickle cell test, and an examination for parasites, if indicated. The hospital repeated these tests and other more complicated procedures, but doing our own laboratory work was considered a part of our training. We used time that might have been better spent in the library, but early on we learned that relatively simple laboratory tests often obviated the need for more complex and expensive tests.

After we finished the initial workup, we read, read, read, preparing for student ward rounds. Generally, these were conducted by the chairman of the department and were awe inspiring because of his erudition and because of our fear. We had mixed emotions. We wanted to hear our patients discussed and to give our impressions, but we were terrified of having missed something. It seemed that one major teaching technique was to expose the medical student who had failed to elicit an important historical fact or had missed a pertinent physical finding. This type of teaching has not changed in fifty years. Many outstanding teachers are still hams and prima donnas, and the medical students are often the unwitting victims of the scenarios. The experience is indelibly imprinted and the individual rarely misses the same thing twice. The most powerful learning must undoubtedly be from one's mistakes, especially those aired in a big hospital ward.

While I was learning about medical care in a large public hospital, I had an unexpected opportunity to work with private patients in a different setting. Billy McCaw, who was now an extern at Baker Memorial Hospital, told me that there was an opening for another extern at Baker. An extern, usually a senior medical student, lived in the hospital, performed histories and physicals, wrote daily progress notes and assisted in the operating room. In exchange, the extern received room, board, uniforms, and laundry. I leapt at the chance to apply for the position, for I was having difficulty living on the money I had borrowed from Dr. Guignard. Letters written to my mother during these years reveal my dire straits. In one letter I was asking to borrow ten dollars to eke out my junior year. The possibility of working at Baker looked like pie in the sky.

When I went to see the Drs. Baker, they told me that they had never had a woman extern so they didn't have living quarters for one, but I could have the job if I was willing to live in the hospital attic. There were several regular bedrooms in the attic with ceilings and big windows, but these were occupied by nurses. My quarters would be in a vast unfinished loft just off of the elevator shaft. When I was shown the space, it was a nice March day and the temperature was reasonably pleasant. With the optimism and naivete of youth, I said that the arrangements would be fine. I was elated to get the position because I would get to work with more patients and I would be relieved of financial concerns.

Billy McCaw helped me move in. Housekeeping sent up a

hospital bed (with a mattress like a rock), a metal bureau, a work table, and a metal straight chair. We positioned the bed beneath the dormer window and put the table nearby, since this single window afforded the only day light. We rigged up a light bulb hanging from a cord looped over a rafter. The naked bulb hung over the table where I would study. Now I had a small island of light twelve feet square beyond which darkness spread out about twenty feet on either end under the sloping eaves. At times I thought I could hear little creatures scuttling about in the dark recesses. But undaunted, I put up hooks on the wall to hang my clothes, tacked up pictures garnered from throwaway medical magazines, suspended a sheet over the bed to keep overhead dust from falling in my face, and settled in. The next morning, I awoke to the fluttering and cooing of pigeons on my window sill and felt very avant garde, as if I were an artist in Greenwich Village. I had to wait several weeks for the prized white uniforms, because the hospital, of course, had no uniforms for a woman. They weren't even manufactured, so the Bakers gave me an allotment for material and my mother made my white skirts and "barber tops." White shoes, polished daily, and a short white coat with dangling stethoscope completed the uniform.

My experience at Baker was valuable and memorable. There were four externs and we rotated working up new patients and assisting in the operating room. Baker was about a sixty-bed hospital, so at all times, each of us was following ten to fifteen patients. Most mornings I was up before day break assisting at one or two tonsillectomies before I walked or ran the two blocks to classes or to ward rounds at Roper Hospital. When I finished my work there, I went back to Baker to assist in more surgery, to see my patients and to write progress notes. I spent an inordinate amount of time with patients, because, like many idealistic medical students, I felt that I had more concern about them than anybody else, even their private physicians. Ah, the arrogance of youth!

This was a very busy time, going to medical school and working at Baker, but I realized what an unusual clinical opportunity I was having. The experience fifty years ago was very different from what individuals in training have now. We saw infectious diseases that are rare today because of immunization (polio, tetanus, diphtheria). We observed prolonged illness and many deaths due to pneumonia, tuberculosis, syphilis, typhoid fever, and a host of other infections that are readily curable today. Most of the deaths were due to lack of effective therapy; this was the pre-antibiotic era. Sulfonamides were just beginning to become available, but were not effective against many types of bacteria. Also, the early sulfonamides had serious side effects that limited their use in some patients.

Things were not much better in other areas of medicine. The only effective drugs for heart problems were digitalis and a few for the management of cardiac arrhythmias (abnormal heart rhythm). Hypertension was difficult to control with the available methods, and there was no such thing as an intensive care unit (cardiac or otherwise); cardiovascular surgery was in its infancy, but pioneering work was ongoing in many institutions including our own. There was little that could be done for patients with cancer. Individuals with most malignancies had a bleak prognosis. Treatment consisted primarily of surgical removal supplemented, in some cases, by implantation of radium or x-ray therapy. Chemotherapy had not come into being. Doctors had to stand by and watch the inexorable march of the malignant process, doing what they could to alleviate suffering. At Baker I watched a young mother, no older than I, waste away from cervical cancer, her young husband trying to convince her and himself that she was not going to die, but to no avail. In a few months she was dead.

Surgical techniques and post-surgical management were different from those of today. Early ambulation was not the rule. Patients were kept at strict bedrest for days or weeks. As a result, many developed pneumonia or pulmonary embolism. I witnessed the shocking death of a forty-year-old woman ten days post-hysterectomy. I was in the room when she was being dressed to go home. She was sitting on the side of the bed conversing with the nurse and me when she gasped, turned blue, and collapsed. She had suffered a massive pulmonary embolism and was dead within fifteen minutes. I went to my attic room and wept.

Fifty years ago, although medical management and surgical management were clearly different and diagnostic techniques were limited, the underlying principles were the same as they are in medicine today. In medical school, we acquired a solid foundation on which to build and to use the astounding advances that would occur in our lifetime. In addition, when we were in our early training and lacked the tools to cure many patients, we learned a lot about the art of medicine. We learned the importance of listening and being compassionate and supportive of the patients and their families. And we learned the importance of allowing the patient to have a dignified, peaceful death. Today, when there is so much rapid, powerful technology, this art of medicine often gets lost.

Through the summer and fall of 1943, during my last year in medical school, I continued the headlong pace at school and at Baker Hospital. Fortunately, I was not in my attic room very much. In the summer it was a sauna, and all year long, the elevator arrived to bong against the top of the shaft night and day. When it was not in use, it automatically returned just beside my room. When the heat and noise became unbearable, I went down to the porch off the operating room and slept on a stretcher, now called a gurney. In the fall, the attic was a refrigerator and I studied in my Harris tweed coat and gloves, but I was young and vigorous and the views from Baker made up for the discomfort. Through the dormer window over my bed, I looked across a small lake, over the rooftops and slender church steeples to the harbor. In the mists of early morning and late at night I felt as though I were in Paris looking across the "chimney pots" to the Seine.

From the operating room porch on the opposite side of the hospital, the view was very different but equally interesting. Here, one looked out on the Ashley River with the war time traffic of coast guard and inshore patrol boats cruising through the blue water against the background of the marshes, bright green in the summer, golden in the winter. On weekends, I sometimes went down to help the nurses working on the operating room porch, just to enjoy the view and to have some feminine companionship. We dried and dusted rubber gloves and prepared various types of surgical packs for sterilization. We examined surgical instruments meticulously for sharpness and put them aside if there were nicks or other flaws – all of this as I listened to hospital gossip or the latest episodes in the nurses' courtships.

This was pre-television soap opera. Today, I am amused when I see the interest that medical personnel exhibit in watching "General Hospital" and other medical soap operas, reminding me of the "do-it-yourself soaps" we used to enjoy on that operating room porch.

The recreation I enjoyed most during my last year in Charleston was sailing. Ike Furman, one of my classmates, introduced me to this wonderful sport. He had grown up in Charleston and had been sailing since he was a small boy. He was an accomplished sailor and during the summers while in college, he earned money crewing on large sailboats that were being moved up and down the Atlantic coast. We went out on an eighteen-foot boat called a snipe, I think, and Ike taught me the basics. One afternoon when we were docking, we discovered a sailboat submerged in about two feet of water near one of the piers at the municipal yacht basin. We found out that it belonged to a man who was in the service and Ike wrote to him to ask about his plans for the boat. The man replied that the boat, including the sails, had been underwater for over a year and was probably worthless, so Ike could have it if he wanted it. It was a thirty-foot racing scow and Ike couldn't raise it alone nor could he afford any repairs, so he recruited a group of ten senior students, and each of us contributed ten dollars for the salvage operation.

The men managed to get the boat afloat, scraped off the barnacles, and caulked and painted her. Now came the matter of sails. The boat had a gaff rig with a tremendous square sail and a smaller jib sail. The sails were in terrible shape from being in the water and mud. The jib was beyond repair, but Ike, the only real sailor among us, assured us we could manage with only the mainsail. The condition of the mainsail was almost as bad as that of the jib, but we refused to admit it. We hauled it to one of the fraternity houses and spread it out on the big piazza to dry. When it was dry, we examined it for tears. We decided that it would be sailworthy if we cut off the bottom six feet and replaced that part with new canvas. We soon found out that sewing heavy canvas was no small task. It was almost impossible to force a needle through it by hand. We solved that problem by using curved surgical cutting needles appropriated from the operating room. Even so, it took us several days to attach the new piece of sail. Then we needed new ropes. By then our funds were so low, that against our better judgment, we settled for cheap cotton ropes. Eventually, we had the boat outfitted and were ready for her maiden voyage.

She was impressive, and when we raised that tremendous sail it was frightening. There was little wind in the yacht basin, so we sailed out slowly into the river, all of us landlubbers taking orders from Ike. Our speed picked up as we entered the Ashley River, but the real test came when we left the mouth of the river, entered the harbor and began to round the battery. Now it was necessary to tack against the wind – something most of us knew little about. Ike explained that the boom would swing across and we might have to duck. In reality, we had to lie flat because we had made a mistake in making the sail too long. Lying down made things a little difficult for the man at the tiller and for the man handling the sheet rope, but they managed, and we soon got into the rhythm of lying down and letting the sail swing across. We were exhilarated, and using nautical phrases like "coming about" and "hard a-lee," when suddenly things went awry. The wind picked up abruptly and the boat proved her racing heritage. We began to go back and forth across the water at an alarming pace, one minute heading out toward Fort Sumter and the next, coming about and heading for the big rocks piled against the battery's sea wall. People walking along the battery were leaning on the iron railing watching this unusual display. Some people even stopped their cars and got out to watch. Each time, as we neared the battery and made a last-minute turn, narrowly avoiding a collision, there was a cheer from the amused onlookers. We were too frightened to be embarrassed. We were concentrating on survival. That boat needed a jib, and in a strong wind, Ike could hardly steer her with only the rudder. Fate and the rotten sail saved us. Suddenly, a strong gust of wind hit the sail and there was a loud rending sound. The sail split from the very top down to the attachment of the new section and began flapping dolefully in the breeze. We lowered the tatters and drifted while we waited for the Coast Guard to discover our plight and haul us in. We thought it a grand adventure.

That was the first of several adventures (or misadventures) on that ill-fated boat. Somehow we patched her up and went out again. Our last sail was around Thanksgiving when the air and the water were pretty chilly. I remember that I was wearing my raincoat. We sailed merrily out into the Ashley, but just as we were opposite the Coast Guard station, the wind became very strong and we heeled over dangerously. Ike yelled, "Let out the sheet!" This meant letting out the sail to slow us down. Unfortunately, the cotton rope had swollen when it got wet and wouldn't slide through the pulley to let out the sail, so over we went. I can remember thinking, as I saw the wide deck coming down on top of me, "Get clear of the boat, don't get caught in the ropes!" Then the grey green water closed over my head. Dragged down by my raincoat, I sank like a rock, but frantic kicks brought me up along side the overturned boat to join my companions who were clinging to the side. There we stayed until once again the Coast Guard came to get us. This time, our rescuers were in a boat with high sides. The sailors let down a rope with a loop on one end. We put our feet into this and they flapped us up on deck like dead fish. That was the last time I saw our sailboat. I don't remember what we did with her. Maybe we gave her to another group of naive landlubbers in the class that followed us.

Our class was to graduate just before Christmas in 1943, and I was proceeding along confidently until early in October when I was summoned to the office of Dr. Kelley, the Chairman of the Department of Internal Medicine. I entered on rubber legs. Dr. Kelley was a stern, cold man, and the verdict was swift and sure. He asked, "Do you want to graduate with your class in December?" I assured him fervently that I did. Then he said, "Well, you won't unless you give up your job and get to studying!" That afternoon I turned over my Baker responsibilities to the other externs and went back to room alone in the quiet place where I had lived before my Baker sojourn. And I studied!

The week that we graduated there was a unique occurrence in Charleston. There was a heavy snow that lasted for two days. The park at the battery with its old oaks and palmettos was white against the sea. It was incredibly, surrealistically lovely, and I realized how much I was going to miss this beautiful city and the wonderful years I had spent here.

Graduation day arrived – the day we had been waiting for for three and one-half work-filled years. We graduated at high noon in a ceremony less formal than usual. We didn't wear caps and gowns because all but three members of the class were in uniform and would receive their commissions as officers simultaneously with receiving their diplomas. Nor was the music traditional. The processional was not something dignified and solemn like "Pomp and Circumstance." We came in to a jazzed-up version of "Let's Remember Pearl Harbor" belted out by a small orchestra heavy on the bass fiddle. After listening to a brief address, we walked across the stage and received our long-awaited M.D. degrees, and then took the solemn Hippocratic Oath. We were doctors! There were wings on my feet!

All of my family came to graduation except my brother, who was away in the service. Even my father was there. He was still having mental problems and exhibiting erratic behavior, so I was apprehensive that he might embarrass himself and all of the family, but he acted appropriately and I was very touched when he gave me a small monetary present that he could ill afford. My family and I spent a happy afternoon in Charleston, none of us quite believing that I was a doctor, and then they left for home.

That night, Marion Davis, a close friend and one of my classmates and I went for a walk on the battery. We watched as the fog rolled in obliterating Fort Sumter and shrouding the naval ships as it laid a blanket of white over the water. Marion said, "Take a good look, Dukes. This is the prettiest thing you will see for a long time." He was right. The next day I left for Columbia for the Christmas holidays before starting my internship in North Carolina, and I never saw a vision so beautiful for many years.

The years in medical school were a pivotal period for me in two ways. They gave me a sound basis for beginning a life in medicine, and they helped me build self esteem. The constancy of Billy McCaw's love for me, my romance with Tucker, my deep friendship with Joe, and the warm support of my classmates made me realize that I was feminine and attractive and that I liked being a girl. Yes, I still felt like a girl. When I graduated, I was not quite twenty-two and I still needed a lot of maturing to become an independent woman. It was not long in coming, though, because internship is a very maturing process!

Chapter 5

Internship and Marriage

WHEN I LEFT SOUTH CAROLINA to intern at North Carolina Baptist Hospital in Winston-Salem, I was unaware that I was entering a period of major change in my life. My plans were to specialize in obstetrics and gynecology, to remain single at least until my training was finished, and then to return to South Carolina to practice OB-Gyn with Kathleen Riley, my roommate during my freshman year in medical school. None of these things happened. During the next three years, I changed my specialty to pediatrics, got married, and never went back to South Carolina to practice.

North Carolina Baptist Hospital was the teaching hospital for Bowman Gray School of Medicine. I had applied there because it offered a two-year rotating internship. Although I planned to specialize in Obstetrics and Gynecology, I wanted to have a general background in medicine before narrowing down. In fact, this was the norm; in 1944, most doctors took a rotating internship before entering specialty training. I would spend my first year in obstetrics, gynecology, and minor surgery, the second in internal medicine and pediatrics. During the first year I would receive room, board, uniforms and laundry, but no salary. This, too, was the norm for the forties. Today hospitals woo medical school graduates with good salaries and numerous "perks" in order to fill their residency slots. During World War II, hospitals had rigid quotas. Some hospitals were required to reduce the number of their house staff positions by as much as two-thirds of their prewar number, so it was considered a privilege to work in a good hospital, either teaching or non teaching. There was no stipend at teaching hospitals and a pittance at those hospitals not associated with medical schools. The more prestigious the hospital, the less the recompense. Anyway we were all in the same boat and accepted this situation with reasonable equanimity. Because women were not subject to the draft, many hospitals began accepting women for internships for the first time, and others that had allowed no training for women beyond the internship year now permitted them to stay additional years for specialty training.

Looking back, the medical school years were my salad days and the house officer years (internship and residency) were the maturing ones. Gone were the fun-filled days in a wartime seaport. Gone was the support of classmates and friends. Now I was really on my own, but without apprehension. I was too naive to realize how tough it would be.

I arrived in Winston-Salem on New Year's Day, 1944, after an all-day train ride in a coach crowded with soldiers, many of them sitting on suitcases in the aisles. I arrived, but my luggage didn't. After searching at the station and filling out a form for lost luggage, I decided that since I had never been to Winston-Salem and didn't know how to catch a bus to the hospital, I would take a cab. This was a serious decision, since it meant invading my precious eighteen dollars that was to last me for the next nine months. But again, I wasn't worried. Everybody knew that interns didn't have any money. All my real needs would be supplied by the hospital.

I entered the hospital, found the administrative office and, with the assurance of my brand new M.D. degree, expected a warm welcome. Suddenly I had my first taste of what it would be like to be an intern, especially a woman intern. When I introduced myself and inquired about quarters, I was greeted with "Oh, you're a woman! The internship and residency committee didn't tell us. We don't have any quarters for women." Next I asked about uniforms only to hear that there were no uniforms, although on my application I had filled in the lines about my measurements, thinking that the hospital would provide them. Again I heard, "We didn't know you were a woman and we don't have any uniforms for women." After one of the secretaries made a series of telephone calls, I was told that I could spend the night in the room of a nurse who was out of town. Then I asked whether I should report to someone in the Ob-Gyn Department. To my dismay the answer was, "No, you're a day late. You were supposed to be here this morning and you've missed orientation. You'll just have to see the chief resident at seven o'clock in the morning." With these douses of cold water, I began to learn two important facts: there is nothing lower than an intern and holidays in a hospital are just like any other days. Be there!

The next morning I reported to the chief resident who turned out to be a big, handsome, arrogant Yankee. On this first day he gave me a severe lecture about being late and about not being in uniform. Then he informed me that along with the other Ob-Gyn intern, I would be on call every other night and every other weekend for the next nine months. Weekends off, meant from Saturday noon until seven A.M. on Monday. There would be no vacation. He reminded me that the term for internship had been reduced from a year to nine months to allow male physicians to enter the service as quickly as possible, but he assured me that the training would not be reduced; the time off would be reduced and the work load increased.

I didn't mind all his barking commands, because everybody was in the same boat and I felt I was merely doing my part for my country; but I did, however, mind his next remarks. He told me that because I was late, I would work five out of the next seven nights, and that there was no place for me to sleep when I was on call. I agreed that I couldn't sleep in the men's call room, but was shocked at his suggestion for alternate sleeping arrangements. He said, "You can sleep on one of the beds in the labor room." I managed not to answer back but my reaction was, "You must be crazy. I'm not sleeping in there with all those screaming women. I'll find some other place. You can count on it, Buddy!"

So I went to work, miserably hot in my wool dress, comfortable only when I donned a scrub dress to go into the delivery or operating suites. In those days, scrub clothes were permitted only in those two areas; they were strictly forbidden elsewhere in the hospital. When we left the delivery or operating suite we had to be in starched white uniforms and polished shoes. My spirits were very low. I had forgotten how low until I read a sad letter my mother had saved.

Monday night
Dear Mother,

Things are still pretty much of a mess but they're slowly straightening out. So many adverse things have happened that I've been about ready to come home 3 or 4x but this is one time I can't come. I've spent the night a different place every night since I've been here. Tonight I'm actually in mine and the other girl intern's room. It is quite small and has as furniture 2 iron beds, 1 bureau, 2 straight chairs. We still can't unpack at all. We're gonna strike for another bureau, some book shelves and possibly a table. We have an awful setup. We're living upstairs over a doctor and his family. We have to go thru their living room to get in and out and the woman believes in locking up the damned place despite the fact that we have no keys. I'm afraid that I'm gonna be very unpleasant soon.

I spend every other night in the hospital and every other weekend. This weekend I have an extra night to put in so I'll be on the floor on call Tues. night, Wed. night, Fri. night, Sat. night, Sunday night. I reckon I'll like the work but it is too much responsibility for me. I'm the only intern on the service, and therefore, have to run the whole business. Every other night I run Ob and Gyn. I'm the only doctor up there and I'm responsible for getting in touch with the others when I think it necessary. Right now it's driving me crazy but I guess I'll get used to it.

When you send my pkg., send as many coat hangers as you can spare. I have none. Also send those other uniforms. I'm gonna use them and get a refund. I have to have a laundry bag. I shall try to get them to give me one.

Hurrah, only one bright spot in my day. I got off an hour & went to the bus station and found my suitcase. It was wonderful to brush my teeth and change underclothes & stockings for the first time since leaving Columbia. I couldn't wash the pants & hose I had on because I was on call all the time.

Janie, the other woman intern (she is in pediatrics) and I alternate getting homesick. She cheers me up, then I cheer her up. We see very little of each other, however, due to our widely divergent hours and locations in the hospital. She's from Penn. & studied med. at Yale. We went to a med meeting together tonight.

She hasn't moved over yet tonight but is staying in the nurses' home. I had to move because it looked like my only chance.

Right now I must retire.

Love,
Martha

P.S. I want to come home but I won't!

Fifty years ago there were many differences in internships from those today, but one thing has remained the same: there was, and is, nothing more pathetic than interns on new terrain. They don't know how to get anything done or where to find anything, such as the laundry, the mail room, the record room, and the laboratories, and there is little time to find out. We were thrown into the maelstrom of work, taking responsibility for patients for the first time. When we were medical students, we thought we knew just what the house officers should do, but now that we were writing the orders, it was frightening. Fortunately, the interns were under the supervision of a second-year person.

There was a strict hierarchy then as there is today. At the base of the pyramid were the medical students, the next tier consisted of the interns, then came the assistant residents, and finally the chief resident reported to the head of the department and to the attending physicians. There was never any doubt about the chain of command in the operating and delivery suites, at the bedside rounds, on entering the elevator, or walking down the hall. The leader walked in front and his entourage followed according to rank.

Nobody was ever more homesick than I was. During the day and well after dark, I was all right, but at twilight homesickness came down over me like a black cloud. I wasn't homesick for my family. I missed Charleston and my classmates. I looked out of the hospital window to see bleak wintry hills and bare trees, not the sea and wheat-colored marshes, not green palmettos and live oaks festooned with moss. When I went to dinner, I couldn't swallow because the lump in my throat was too big. There were no friends to share complaints and laughter. My roommate and I rarely saw each other because our schedules were too divergent. I had entered a world of conservative male interns, most of whom had gotten their medical training at Bowman Gray and had done their undergraduate work at Wake Forest College, a strict Baptist school. They were very different from the "live-it-up" men at the medical college in Charleston, and when I ventured a funny or irreverent remark, they looked at me as if I were a weird, unknown species. However, despite my loneliness, I rapidly came to realize that I had made a wise decision in selecting the Bowman Gray School of Medicine-North Carolina Baptist Hospital program, because of the close interaction between the faculty, house officers, and medical students.

In 1944, Bowman Gray School of Medicine (physically connected to North Carolina Baptist Hospital) was only three years old. It had formerly been a two-year school at Wake Forest College in the little town of Wake Forest, North Carolina; the students had to transfer to other schools for the last two years. When Winston-Salem's city fathers (including Bowman Gray and R. J. Reynolds) supported its move to Winston-Salem, it was renamed and became a four-year school with many innovative ideas. Dr. Tinsley Harrison, the well known internist, came from Vanderbilt to be the first dean, and the chairmen of the various departments were recruited from Johns Hopkins, Harvard, and other outstanding schools. They were all young, vigorous, and enthusiastic about building a fine school and teaching students and house officers. There was an air of excitement about learning.

Ob-Gyn interns were expected to be everywhere – examining new patients, assisting in deliveries, assisting in Caesarian sections, assisting in gyn surgery, writing progress notes, and dictating discharge summaries in the record room. It rapidly became apparent that the work load was too heavy for the two of us who were interns, so at the end of the first week, the decision was made for two medical students to act as externs and assist us. None of the six medical students who were rotating through the service volunteered, so they decided to toss coins. The two students who lost the toss were assigned to work every other night and every other weekend. One of the students who lost the toss was Ellard Yow, and he was assigned to work with me. Ellard had received his M.D. in December, 1943, from Bowman Gray, but needed to complete the student requirements for Ob-Gyn and Pediatrics, because during his sophomore year he had taken off a quarter to act as an assistant in Physiology. He knew all the ropes and his working with me was a terrific boon. There was only one problem: I couldn't understand his name. Finally, I asked him, "Please, write it for me. I don't want to wake you up at night by calling, 'Hey Boy!'" After I mastered his name, we were all set to work together.

Many important things in our lives are determined by chance. Fate was certainly kind to me, when by the flip of a coin, Ellard and I were brought together. We were congenial from the outset, although he was a few years older than I, and much more mature. I was a naive, provincial, insecure, brash young woman. He was self-assured, quiet and calm, and knew how to get things done. He did his work efficiently, thoroughly, and cheerfully. Neither of us procrastinated. One thing I learned in obstetrics was to do everything as quickly as possible. When a new patient was admitted, we examined her immediately. You never knew when there would be a rush of other admissions, when somebody would have to be delivered, or when some woman would start bleeding and have to have an emergency C-section. We were busy, but occasionally there was a brief lull when we could sit around with the medical students telling stories and laughing.

Ellard and I found that we had mutual interests in literature and music. He had gone to Davidson College where he had a classical education and majored in psychology before deciding to go to medical school. He had a broader education than most of us who had focused on premed. I was especially impressed that he had taken Greek, and that while at Davidson, he had become an accomplished French horn player. We discussed books and music but most of all we shared our love of the sea. I told him my sailing stories and he told me about his adventures on the Pamlico Sound in his father's cabin cruiser.

A week after we began working together, he asked me to go bowling. He didn't know it, but it was my twenty-second birthday and I had been so homesick all day that I accepted with enthusiasm. I was astonished when he arrived in a big Packard, his mother's, and he was surprised when I came to the door in a maroon velveteen swing skirt, a soft rose-colored sweater, and long pearls. He blurted out, "You don't look the same in clothes!" That was the first of many nights together. On most of the nights when we were not working side by side, we dated. When I asked him later why he asked me out that first night, he answered, "You weren't like any girl I had ever known, and you told such funny, crazy stories that I wanted to see what you were like." I thought, "Well, maybe Mother had a point with her, 'Have the courage to be different.'"

By the end of the first two weeks, I was feeling much better. I had settled into a routine and had appropriated a vacant hospital room to use on my nights on call. The administration was not happy about it, but did not oust me. I was increasingly interested in Ellard and he in me. My heart raced when I saw him coming down the hall with his red hair, freckled face, and bouncing walk expressing enthusiasm at every step. I was very attracted to him and deeply impressed by what a wonderful doctor he was already at the age of twenty-five.

We worked well together and one particular night stands out in my mind. On this night there was a woman who had no private doctor and no money, so she became the responsibility of the house staff. She was in labor with her third child and no complications were expected, so I was to deliver her without the assistance of the resident. Of course, if she developed problems, I was to call him. Things went smoothly until the patient was in the delivery room. Then all of a sudden, when it was too late to call for help, there was trouble. The baby's head was large and the woman's perineum bulged alarmingly. She pushed and pushed to no avail, and I became alarmed that she might have a serious tear of the vagina. I decided that I would have to do an episiotomy (an incision to enlarge the vaginal opening), rather than risk a tear. I had seen many episiotomies and they looked easy, so I asked the anesthetist to put the patient to sleep. Then I proceeded to make a nice, clean incision and delivered a strapping baby boy. Now came the task of repairing the episiotomy. I was sitting on a stool at the end of the table ready to sew, and Ellard was standing just behind me looking over my right shoulder. Much to my dismay, the incision gaped open and all of the layers of tissue flowed together. They had to be sutured in layers; mucous membrane, muscle, and finally skin. The divisions were hard to visualize, but I started on what I thought was mucous membrane. When it was time for muscle, the situation was even more confusing. I whispered to Ellard, "I can't do it." He whispered back, "Keep going, keep going, you're doing fine." At that moment, I thought, "This is the man for me." He was so calm and inspired so much confidence, that I continued to suture and at last finished as well as I could. It was not a very good looking job, and I was really worried because I was afraid I had done it wrong. After we left the delivery room and were alone, I confided to Ellard, "I'm afraid I'm in big trouble. I'm afraid I've created a third sex."

The next morning when we went on staff rounds (the full entourage, including the chairman of the department) examining the breasts, palpating the uterus, and inspecting the perineum of every woman on the service, I was sweating with apprehension. To my amazement, my handiwork looked perfect and I drew a big sigh of relief. Nature is a wonderful thing and the body has a remarkable ability to repair itself.

Looking back, that night in the delivery room was a turning point in my life because I realized how supportive and dependable Ellard was. Later I had many opportunities to see Ellard make wise decisions and inspire confidence, but that experience was of special significance, because it was the first time that I realized how important he was to me.

From then on our romance blossomed. I'll never know how. We were so bad looking in the operating and delivery rooms. Often my hair was in bobby pins under the green scrub cap and the scrub dresses I wore were so ill fitting that I was teased about my "Hattie Carnegie models." Ellard looked even worse. He was concerned about control of infection, so he wore his cap low on his forehead and down over his ears. Most of the men wore them at a jaunty angle, but not Ellard. But love conquered all and beauty was in the eye of the beholder. On the rare occasions when we were in the scrub room alone, dressed in these outlandish garbs, soapsuds dripping from our elbows, we would work in a quick embrace and kiss!

Now life was really looking much brighter, but at the end of my first month as an intern, the bubble burst. I was notified that I would spend the next two months at a branch of the county hospital eighteen miles out in the country. When I protested, "But that is not in my contract," I learned that the matter was not negotiable. Every rotating intern had to spend two months in this little hospital. So off I went in the middle of a cold, bleak February. I felt as if I were being sent to Siberia, and both Ellard and I were upset. This meant that we would have real difficulty seeing each other because, due to gas rationing, he was allotted only three gallons a month and that was not many miles in a Packard. But youth is resourceful, and we would soon find a way to be together.

The hospital was a small cottage-type facility where medical care was provided to the rural indigent – all ages, all problems. The medical staff consisted of Dr. James O'Neill, an assistant professor of surgery from the medical school, a handful of nurses, and me. We took care of the elderly, handled pediatric problems, delivered babies, and performed minor surgery. Here under supervision, I did my first appendectomies, minor Gyn surgery, set simple fractures, and treated all manner of wounds.

Adjacent to the hospital were two units of the state prison system (one for women and one for men), and the inmates received their medical care by our making house calls in the prison. I dreaded to be called to the men's unit, and usually Dr. O'Neill took care of these calls, but when he was in Winston-Salem operating, I had to go. The most common problem was acute urinary retention due to a urethral stricture. This necessitated dilation of the urethra with sounds, a series of evil looking curved steel rods, starting with the smallest in diameter and progressing to the larger sizes. When the dilation was accomplished, one could then catheterize the patient. The prison always seemed dark and foreboding, and I was always frightened despite being escorted by a big, black guard. Amazingly, although the procedure was very painful, none of the prisoners ever became violent. The pain from their distended bladders was so severe, that they welcomed the relief and were almost pathetically grateful. It didn't take me long, though, to know that I didn't want to be a urologist.

Dr. O'Neill, the nurses, and I all lived in pleasant rooms in the hospital and ate in a home-like dining room. Often in the mornings I ate alone with a hefty black woman prisoner cooking my breakfast to order. One morning I ventured a question, "Mamie, what are you in here for?" She replied, "Lawd, I didn't do nothing wrong. I just cut a big buck nigger that was m'lestin me. I was jus sittin on de curb mining my own bizness and havin my top and bottom (ale and whiskey) when dis no count nigger come up and grab me by the front of my new dress. He toe it down the front. Dat jus hep me to get to my knife quicker and I giv him a good slash! Dat's why I'm heayar. What you want for breakfast?" I answered quickly, "Anything, Mamie, just anything." After that I made no special demands or had any complaints. Whatever Mamie served, I ate with a big smile.

It wasn't long before I found that one of my duties at the county hospital offered a way to see Ellard. I had to make emergency house calls all over the county, sometimes extending across the Virginia border. For these calls I drove the ambulance, a converted bread truck equipped with flashing lights and a siren. Since I didn't know the area, it was difficult for me to find patients living on dark, unmarked, country dirt roads. On many calls, unbeknownst to Dr. O'Neill, I telephoned Ellard and went in to Winston-Salem to pick him up, serving two purposes. We got to be together, and he helped me find the patients. One of us drove, and since there was only one seat in the ambulance, the other sat on an upended apple crate. Then, of course, I had to drive Ellard back to Winston-Salem, and we extended the trip with a little courting. Dr. O'Neill occasionally expressed some concern about how that woman intern could use so much gas and why it took her so long to make calls.

One night Ellard had to work, and I had to make a house call that I shall never forget. I followed the directions given me by a family member calling on the phone at a filling station. "You come five miles on to Mr. Jones' house, then you passes a two-story white house and dat ain' it. You turns at the corner by the store wid de Esso sign and come till you see a fork in de road. You takes the lef fork tru the cornfield and dat's us." When I arrived at the small unpainted house about 1:00 A.M., a black man was waiting on the porch. He showed me through the living room that was filled with family and friends. I went into the small, dimly lit bedroom to see the familiar face of Sam Riley.

Sam had been in the hospital two weeks before, when I treated him for burns he received when he had a seizure and fell into the fireplace. He told us he had been having "spells" for a number of years. While he was in the hospital, I had tried to do a good physical examination, but he was six feet tall, weighed well over two hundred pounds, and was belligerent and combative, and although the orderly restrained him, I couldn't obtain a reliable blood pressure reading. He got out of bed against orders and several times fell on the floor with seizures. His family verified his history of having seizures for some time and told us that he had been diagnosed as having epilepsy, so after his burns improved we did no further evaluation and he was discharged from the hospital.

When I saw Sam on this house call, I was shocked. He was a different man. He appeared to have shrunken since the last time I had seen him. He was able to tell me that he had gone to a barbecue picnic on the previous day and afterwards had developed severe abdominal pain, diarrhea, and vomiting. Now he looked terribly ill, his pulse was weak, and he was having trouble breathing. His blood pressure was very low, indicating shock. I had no idea what to do. I looked in the medical bag and found some adrenalin, but before giving him anything, I felt that I needed to tell the people in the living room how things stood. I explained, "Sam is terribly sick and I'm not sure I can save him but I'm going to give him this shot and then try to get him to the hospital." I ventured nervously back to the bedside, drew up a small dose of adrenalin in the syringe and injected it. Sam drew one gasping breath, foam ran out of his mouth and he fell back dead.

I was terribly shaken, but I knew I had to face that room full of friends and family and I had to try to get permission for an autopsy. As house officers, we had been indoctrinated about the importance of obtaining autopsies for the sake of the family and to increase medical knowledge. So I pled with the family and they agreed to the autopsy. But then came the matter of getting Sam's body onto the stretcher and into the ambulance. All the men demurred, one stating, "I ain't having no truck wid de dead," but finally I prevailed. So, at five o'clock in the morning, very tired and shaken, but proud of myself, I drove up to the morgue at the hospital in Winston-Salem.

Two weeks later I had less reason for pride. Sam's case was chosen for the weekly pathological conference and I went in to Winston-Salem to attend. This was a superb teaching conference held in a large circular amphitheater. All the faculty attended, and student and house officer attendance was mandated. A house officer presented the case and a senior faculty member discussed it. Several days before the conference, they received a resume of the case and were prepared to discuss the differential diagnosis. This time Dr. Tinsley Harrison was the faculty member, a dynamic teacher and showman. Sitting high in the amphitheater, I was feeling very self-satisfied. I must have brought in a fascinating and difficult case if the mighty Dr. Harrison was to be the discussant.

The house officer presented the case and listed his diagnoses in order of probability. Then Dr. Harrison gave a brilliant analysis of the case including an acerbic remark about there being no blood pressure recorded on the hospital chart. He stressed the need for this information because his primary diagnosis was pheochromocytoma, a tumor of the adrenal that causes elevation of the blood pressure.

Next the pathologist gave his postmortem findings. This was a moment he savored, because he enjoyed the upsmanship of reporting a diagnosis unsuspected by the clinician. He announced that the patient had a rare condition, Whipple's Disease. He went on to describe the symptoms: abdominal pain, diarrhea, weight loss, and joint pain. He concluded these remarks by saying there was no treatment and it was often fatal. I felt good and very relieved. It didn't matter about the blood pressure. I had obtained an autopsy on a patient with a rare disease and I couldn't have saved his life. I even felt exonerated about not having taken his blood pressure.

But the pathologist wasn't through. He continued, "The patient had another finding that may have led to his death. He did have a pheochromocytoma." My heart sank. I had heard about this relatively rare tumor. I knew that it secreted epinephrine (adrenalin) causing hypertension, damage to the heart and kidneys, and frequently "fainting spells." I had given a patient who had excessive levels of adrenalin in his blood a dose of adrenalin! At that time few cases had been described in the literature, but that didn't save me. Dr. Harrison rose to his feet, "Where is the intern who took care of this patient?" Trembling, knees almost buckling I stood up.

Dr. Harrison fixed me with beady eyes, "Why was there no blood pressure recorded on the hospital chart?"

"I couldn't take one, because the patient was so belligerent."

"What did you think you were treating when you saw him at his home?"

"I didn't know, " I replied.

"Why did you give him adrenalin?"

"Because it was the only emergency drug in the bag."

I felt terrible about the patient and also about having my ignorance exposed in front of the whole amphitheater of doctors and students. Later, though, some of the faculty reassured me that the small amount of adrenalin I had administered could not have altered the course of Sam's illness. My peers, the other house officers, were less kind. After that when I was deliberating about how to treat a patient, they enjoyed asking, "Why don't you try some adrenalin, Martha?"

For forty years, I looked for pheochromocytoma in every patient with unexplained hypertension or seizures, and although I saw patients whom other doctors had diagnosed as having this tumor, I never found one myself. But I became adamant about blood pressures being recorded on the chart. Once, years later when I was the attending physician, I heard a resident whisper, "Here she comes. You sure as hell better have a blood pressure on the chart!"

Finally, my two months of exile were over and I went back to my duties on the Ob-Gyn service at the Baptist Hospital. In the meantime, Ellard had completed his medical school requirements and was a full-fledged intern in internal medicine. Now he was assured of nine months of training before going into the service, and we began to talk seriously about marriage. His proposal was hardly romantic. He said, "Either we are going to have to get married or stop going together. This working every other night and dating the next is exhausting." He added, "But you have to choose between me and South Carolina. I don't plan to live there and you have to be willing to go wherever I go." That gave me pause but it was a short pause, because I was deeply in love and wanted to get married. When I was dating during my medical school days, I had repeatedly asserted that I wouldn't consider getting married until I finished my internship and residency training, but now, I completely lost my resolution. Like many young couples, Ellard and I were caught up in the war-time urgency. The war was raging in Europe and the Pacific, and men and women were getting married at an earlier age than was usual because of the imminent threat of separation and possible death of the men. We wanted to get married as soon as possible.

Once engaged, we didn't see each other as frequently, for soon thereafter the other Ob-Gyn intern who alternated duty with me quit. He'd heard about a new bill, the G.I. bill, that would pay servicemen to go back into training after their tours of duty, and he went into the service so that he would be paid when he came back into an internship. At least that was the interpretation of the other house officers. Perhaps it was patriotism, or perhaps he thought the work load was too great. Whatever the reason, he left and then there was me. This, of course, created a serious hardship for me. I worked almost continuously from the middle of April until the middle of May, going to my room only for clean clothes. Ellard, too, was working hard on internal medicine, and the time we spent together was mostly in the doctor's lounge. This was in the days before beepers, and we had to stay where we could hear the speaker, "Dr. Yow, Dr. Yow, Dr. Ellard Yow, Dr. Dukes, Dr. Dukes, Dr. Martha Dukes," but we managed to work in a fair amount of necking anyway, grabbing up a newspaper and pretending to read when any of the other doctors came in. One day one of the private doctors said, "You two have been reading the same paper for a week."

One good thing about having such a full life was that I wasn't homesick any more. I was just working day and night as hard as I could, but in spite of this I could never please the chief resident. I couldn't decide whether he hated all women, hated women doctors, or just hated me. Certainly, he was disrespectful to women. He referred to all women patients as "gals" and felt free to slap nurses on the fanny. Fortunately he didn't slap me, or I might have slapped him back. He just stayed on my back and refused to understand why I couldn't be three places at once. One Sunday we had a febrile patient and he had me paged every hour to see whether I was watching her and to ask me her temperature. The intimation was, of course, that I couldn't be trusted to do my job. This was my first significant experience with discrimination and harassment.

Then I committed the ultimate indiscretion. I asked for a week off to get married. I didn't ask the chief resident, because I knew he would refuse. I went over his head and asked the chairman of the department. He said, of course, that I had been doing double duty and that not only could I have the week off, but he wanted to come to the wedding. Ellard's chairman, Dr. Tinsley Harrison, was much less enthusiastic. He was of the school that didn't approve of interns being married, and he told Ellard that he was making a big career mistake to marry that "woman intern." He even called me in and tried to talk me out of it. He insisted that I would jeopardize Ellard's career, but expressed no concern at all about mine. Since I couldn't see how being married would damage either of our careers, he didn't succeed in dissuading me, but he did give Ellard a week off.

How could we afford to get married? I had about ten dollars to my name, but Ellard had five hundred dollars that he had saved from his army pay during medical school. In addition, the hospital agreed to give each of us nine dollars per month as a housing allowance. So we found a big room with shared bath in a private home, in walking distance of the hospital. We would continue to have all of our meals at the hospital, so we thought we could manage very well. On May 20, four months after we met, we were married in a small chapel wedding, and then were off to the coast to spend a glorious week boating on the Pamlico Sound.

Chapter 6

I Almost Quit Medicine

WHEN WE RETURNED TO Winston-Salem, I was calmer about the work load at the hospital because Ellard and I were happy together, and I thought I was tolerating the chief resident's badgering better. But before long I was more exhausted than I realized and was losing weight. I now weighed one hundred eight pounds, and at five feet-eight I looked emaciated. One night when I came home after sixty hours on duty, Ellard asked me some question about my future plans for training, reminding me that the time to apply for an assistant residency the next year was running out. With that, I burst into tears. The second half of the two-year rotating internship (internal medicine and pediatrics) had been discontinued because of the urgent need for doctors in the service, so the logical course for me was to continue in Ob-Gyn. But my internship in Ob-Gyn had been so backbreaking, so crushing to my spirit, that I couldn't face another year of working on that service. I sobbed, "I've made a terrible mistake. I don't like medicine and I don't want to be a doctor!" Ellard was understanding and supportive. He listened sympathetically to my woes and when I had become quieter, told me, "You can quit. Of course, I will support you, but before you quit, why don't you give pediatrics a whirl? Maybe they have a spot and I'll be glad to have you out of that fanny-slapping Ob-Gyn bunch."

Well, of course, I wouldn't really have quit medicine – being a doctor was central to my life. I was just so tired and discouraged that I needed exactly what Ellard provided – a logical alternative to my continuing in Ob-Gyn. Pediatrics had not particularly appealed to me in medical school, but there we had only a brief exposure to working with children, and I really had no concept of the specialty. Ellard's suggestion seemed to be a good course of action. If I liked pediatrics, I would continue, but if later I decided to return to Ob-Gyn, knowledge about infants would be valuable. So the next day I went to see Dr. Robert Lawson, Head of the residency program in Pediatrics.

Dr. Lawson was a big, blond, no-nonsense man who had come to Bowman Gray from Johns Hopkins. He told me that there was a three-month opening for an intern in Pediatrics at the end of my current Ob-Gyn internship, but then there would be a six-month interval when I would have to do something else before continuing in Pediatrics as an assistant resident. That was, if my performance during the first three months on Pediatrics was satisfactory. He told me that I would be on probation, which shocked me (apparently the Ob-Gyn resident had circulated the rumor that I was lazy and a dilettante). In any event, I accepted the three-month offer and made arrangements with the Chairman of Ob-Gyn to be a research fellow in Ob-Gyn for the succeeding six months. By mutual agreement, I was to have no clinical duties, but would assist him in his research.

My rotation as a Pediatric intern was a totally new experience. The patients were interesting and the residents and faculty were dedicated to teaching. The number of patients was small so we were expected to know every detail about each child – not just the present illness, but the growth and development, nutritional status, and the child's relationship to his family. We were given a key to the library so that we could read about the illnesses we were seeing. No matter what time of day or night a patient was admitted, we were required to have read something about his problem before eight o'clock rounds the next morning.

Dr. Lawson became the most important mentor in my medical life. When I started my Pediatric training, he was about thirty-five years old and a dynamo of energy. I remember him on rounds as being in full sail – white coat flying out behind him.

He had a wonderful sense of humor, but when it came to Pediatrics he was all business. He expected us to work hard and to be self reliant, but he was always available when we needed help with a patient. During the day he ran up the stairs to the pediatrics floor from his office (the elevator was too slow for him), and at night, he arrived within the fifteen minutes it took to come from his home. Many nights he worked side-by-side with the house officers taking care of seriously ill children. From him I learned dedication, scientific honesty, and discipline. We observed firm rules of behavior: no leaning on beds; no touching of crib sides unless necessary; and meticulous adherence to isolation and infection control policies. One of the most important rules was that there would be no discussion of patients in the halls or the elevator, because confidentiality was rigidly protected. Dr. Lawson insisted on formality and courtesy between doctors and nurses and on special courtesy and compassion in dealing with families.

I thrived on this routine but I was acutely aware of my probational status. So was Ellard. I think of this as my, "Have you read?" period. When I came home Ellard would greet me with an arm load of books and journals and ask, "Have you read *The New England Journal* this week? There's a good article about meningitis," or "I brought you a book on growth and development from the library." He wanted me to succeed, and we spent many evenings studying and discussing our interesting or difficult cases. In the mornings when I arrived on the Pediatric ward, Dr. Lawson was waiting for me with, "Have you read this book on prematurity? Have you read about the new method of diagnosing cystic fibrosis?" It was a good three months and I enjoyed it. At the end of the time, Dr. Lawson again told me that there was no current opening in Pediatrics, but that I could start an assistant residency in six months. He didn't mention removing the probation, but that didn't bother me because I knew I had done well during my three months as a Pediatric intern.

The interim period of Ob-Gyn research was restful – no nights, no weekends. For the first time in several years I slowed down, got a reasonable amount of sleep, and began to gain back the weight lost during my year of internship. Best of all I began to learn bacteriologic techniques that I would use the rest of my life. My work for Dr. Lock, the Chairman of Ob-Gyn, consisted of studying the bacteriology of the normal vagina, doing library work, and some preliminary writing for him.

Another of my duties was to help Dr. Lock's laboratory assistant in running pregnancy tests. It was long before the days of home kits. Pregnancy tests had to be performed in female rabbits – mean things that kicked and scratched with their sharp claws. We injected urine from the patient into the rabbit's ear vein. Then a few days later, we anaesthetized the rabbit and operated on her to visualize the ovaries. If the patient was pregnant, the hormones in her urine caused the rabbit to ovulate, and we could see the ova on the surface of the ovaries. When I remember this, I hear an old bit of doggerel:

> Tell me, tell, me, little rabbit,
> Does a fertilized egg my womb inhabit?
> Hurry, hurry, little bunny,
> This suspense is not so funny.
> I am sorry, my little dove,
> A fertilized egg comes of thy love,
> Sofa tactics seldom come to naught,
> So before it is too late,
> Try marriage or ergotrate.

I really liked Dr. Lock. He treated me fairly and with respect. I suspect that if the chief resident had not been interposed between us, I would have enjoyed my Ob-Gyn internship and would have continued in that specialty.

When I resumed my Pediatric training as an assistant resident, I was in my element and my work was a pleasure. This was probably the best learning year of my hospital training. I was feeling secure about writing orders, and the interns took care of many of the routine tasks, so that I had time to supervise their work and to really study and think about patients. I still worked every other night and every other weekend, but it was not a hardship. The work load was reasonable, and if all was quiet on midnight rounds, the assistant resident could take calls from home.

Ellard was now an assistant resident, too. He had been selected as one of a limited number of residents who were essential to keep the hospital's teaching program going and who were being trained to provide specialists for the armed services. As a result we had two years together in Winston-Salem after we were married. They were good years. We both enjoyed our work and each of us earned forty dollars a month. We felt so affluent that we moved from our bedroom to an efficiency apartment. The rent was thirty-six dollars a month, but the hospital still gave us eighteen of that. We continued to eat at the hospital, because our ration cards were there and because we couldn't afford the time or money to eat at home. We transformed our unused kitchen space into office space, using the cabinets as files. We even had files under the sink and our marriage license still bears the stains from a leak in the water pipes. Our social life was good. We went to movies, played cards with other house officers and their wives, and Ellard resumed his music, playing his French horn in the North Carolina Symphony, when it performed in our vicinity, and frequently playing in the Moravian brass choir in Old Salem. Each year we had a week off, and of course, spent it on the Pamlico River and Sound going by water to old North Carolina coastal towns.

Our marriage became even more enjoyable as both of us developed an interest in infectious diseases. Here, I should pause to explain the term "infectious diseases." There is the mistaken impression that the term infectious diseases is synonymous with contagious diseases, diseases transmitted from person to person, such as measles, mumps, chicken pox, influenza, and tuberculosis. Contagious diseases are, indeed, infectious diseases, but the field of infectious diseases is much broader, encompassing all disease processes caused by microorganisms (bacteria, viruses, fungi, parasites), including wound and burn infections.

Ellard and I became involved in working with infectious diseases for different reasons. He became a protege of Dr. George Harrell, a professor in the Department of Medicine, who had a major interest in the field and had outfitted a small research lab where he and Ellard did diagnostic work on patients with infections. They began to do special procedures not yet performed routinely in the hospital laboratory, such as testing the sensitivity of bacteria to penicillin, and measuring levels of the drug in blood and other body fluids. The methods were time consuming and cumbersome; however, Dr. Harrell and Ellard worked out refinements to the methods and performed them in all cases in which penicillin seemed indicated.

My interest in infectious diseases came about in a different way. I began working in the lab with Ellard, because such a large percentage of the patients admitted to the pediatric service had infectious diseases. Today most children with infections are managed in outpatient settings before their problems progress and become serious. Fifty years ago, these young patients had to be treated in the hospital, because safe and effective antimicrobial agents were not available for outpatient use. Also, many children had diseases now prevented by immunization. Polio struck mercilessly, and typhoid fever, tuberculosis, tetanus, and diphtheria were often lethal. Meningitis was especially feared, because about ninety percent of patients with the various types of bacterial meningitis died (today, the mortality rate is five percent).

The need for rapid diagnoses in all of these seriously ill children led me to begin taking specimens to Dr. Harrell's lab to study them myself, frequently with Ellard's help. In the research lab, I could experiment with special culture media and check the cultures at more frequent intervals than could be done in the hospital laboratory, making it possible to detect fastidious organisms that required special growing conditions, and to arrive at a specific diagnosis as quickly as possible.

I don't think that my lifelong fascination with infectious diseases was born in that small laboratory, but it was the living out of dreams I had as a teenager reading *Arrowsmith* and *Microbe Hunters*, imagining myself making discoveries like those of Pasteur and Koch. I made no great discoveries, but I got great gratification from influencing patients' outcomes by the work I did in that little lab. Two especially good experiences with young patients are etched in my memory and I am joyful every time I think about them.

Jimmy was a nine-year-old, red-haired, freckled-faced boy from the mountains of North Carolina. When he came to the hospital he had been having intermittent fever for three months, had lost seventeen of his seventy pounds, and was weak and very pale beneath his freckles. He had a history of rheumatic fever at six years of age, and was left with a damaged heart valve. His referring physician felt that the boy had either a recurrence of rheumatic fever or bacterial endocarditis (bacterial infection of the damaged valve).

Within two days, we knew that Jimmy had bacterial endocarditis when we grew large numbers of streptococci from his blood. This was a dreaded diagnosis because, before the advent of penicillin, it was universally fatal. And even though we had penicillin in the mid forties, many patients were not cured because there was such a small amount of penicillin available for an individual patient. In fact, during the war years, the supply of penicillin for civilian use was so limited that hospitals had special committees to decide which patients would receive it and in what amounts.

When Ellard and I tested the penicillin sensitivity of the streptococcus isolated from Jimmy's blood, it was exquisitely sensitive, so the "penicillin committee" allotted 100,000 units of penicillin per day for Jimmy's treatment. This was a generous amount in 1944, but minuscule compared to today's dose of millions of units per day for endocarditis. I was the intern assigned to Jimmy; Jack Reinhart, the chief resident, supervised me; and Dr. Lawson was our staff consultant. The three of us met Jimmy's parents to explain the necessity for intensive, long-term therapy. They agreed because they understood the gravity of the situation. Now we started three weeks of penicillin therapy with Jimmy receiving a painful intramuscular injection every three hours around the clock, the standard method of giving penicillin at that time. The antibiotic was so rapidly excreted in the urine, that it had to be given at frequent intervals in order to be effective.

Blood cultures became negative promptly for as long as we were giving the penicillin, but two days after it was discontinued, they were again positive. Everybody (Jimmy, his parents, the doctors, and the nurses) was discouraged. In the test tube, the streptococcus was easily killed by penicillin, but ridding Jimmy's heart valve of the infection was a different matter. One thing was definite, we weren't going to give up and lose this wonderful boy! Now we had to try some other approach.

We had heard about the administration of penicillin by continuous intravenous drip (the usual way it is given in serious

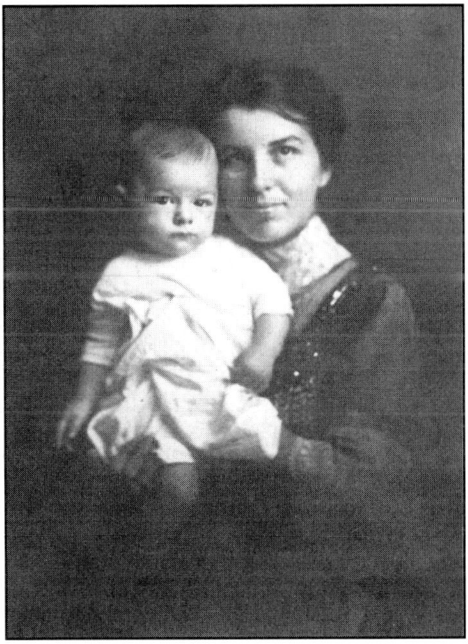

My mother, Volina Ouzts Dukes, age twenty-six, with her first child, my brother, Arthur Dow.

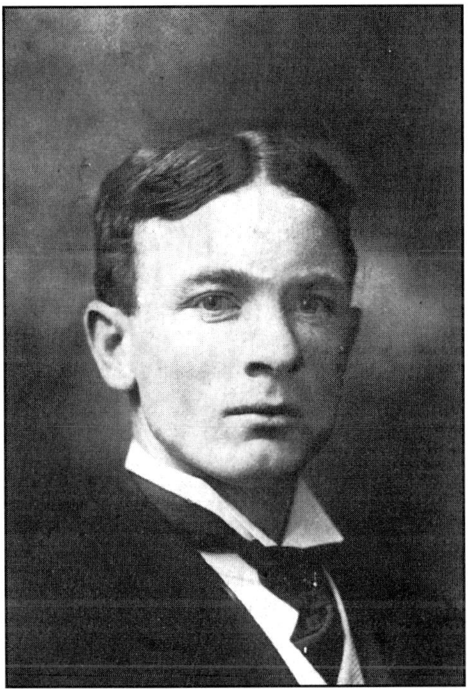

My father, Thomas Edmund Dukes, age thirty-one.

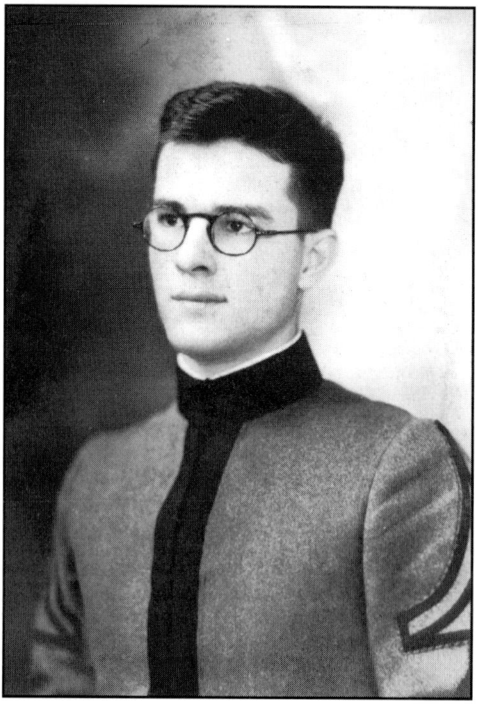

Arthur Dow at The Citadel. He was ten years older than I and always protective and supportive of me.

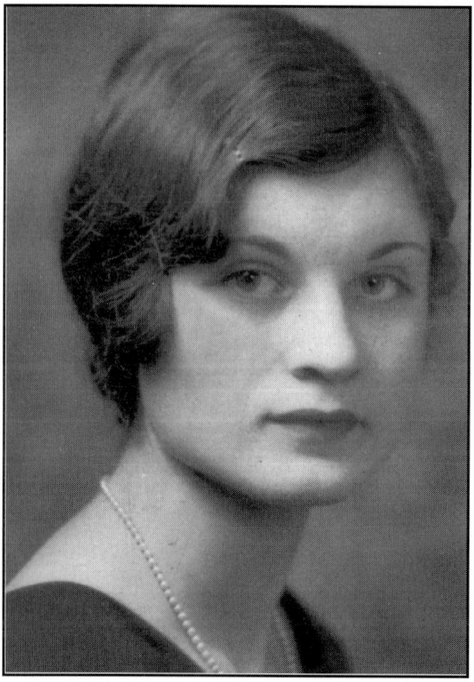

My sister, Catherine, at Lander College in Greenwood. She was eight years my senior and a wonderful role model.

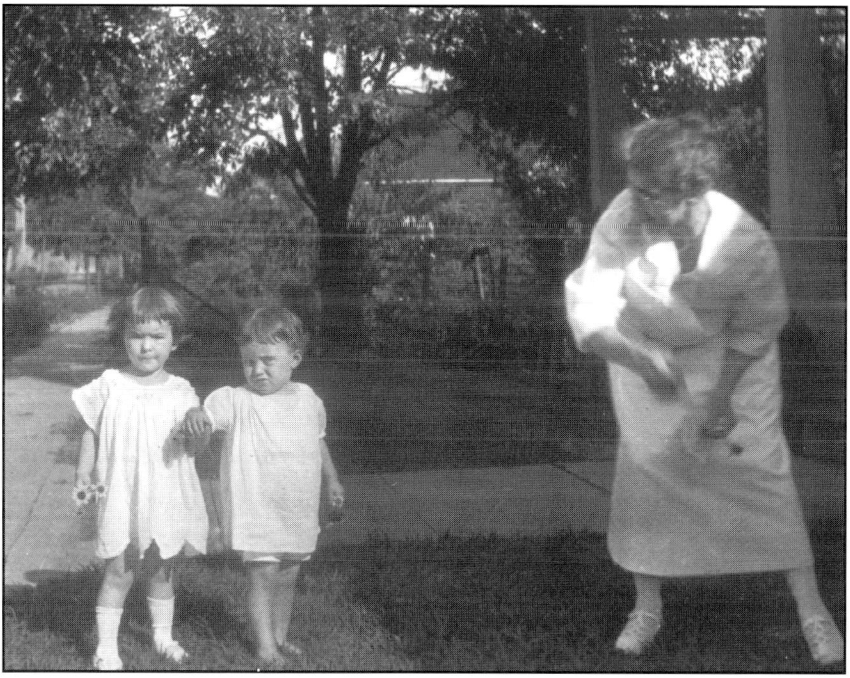

My Aunt Lala tries to get two small girls to pose.
I'm the determined one on the left.

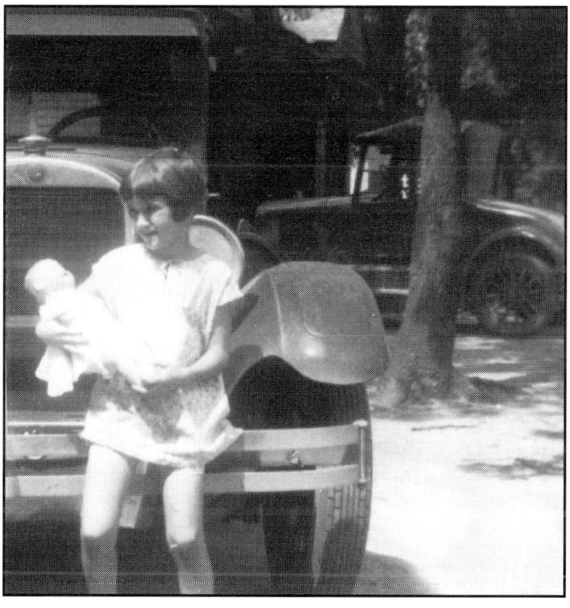

Sometimes I played with dolls.

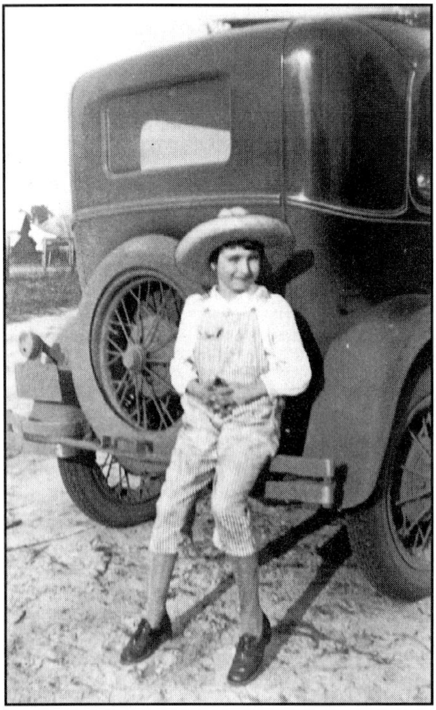

Left:
But I was always prepared for more adventurous activities.

Below:
The Greenwood High School basketball team. I'm holding the ball.

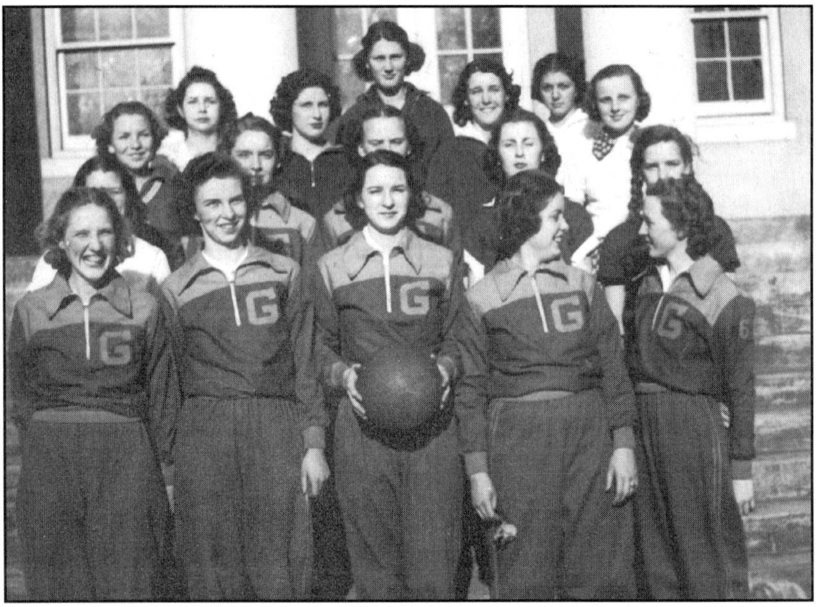

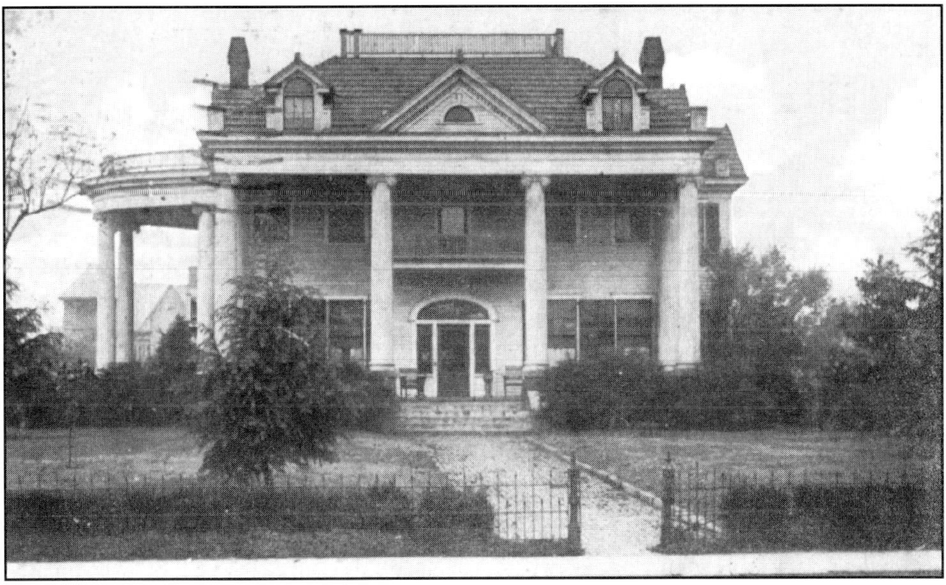

My friend Gee's beautiful home in Greenwood where we exchanged endless confidences.

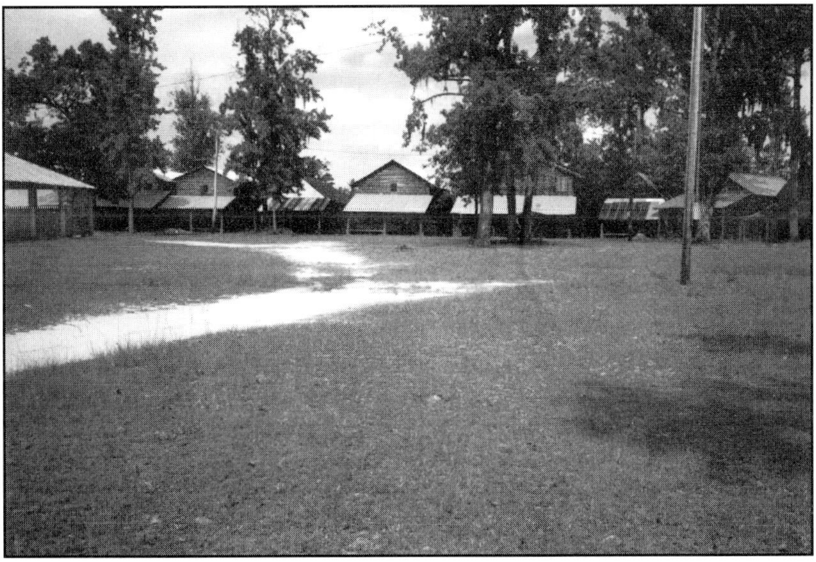

"Tents" at Cattle Creek Campground.
The sandy path was the promenade area.

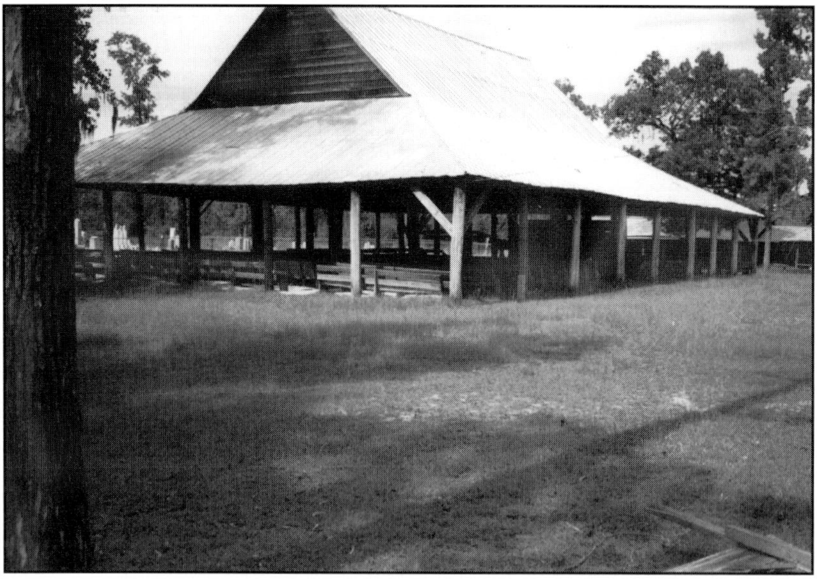

The Tabernacle where services were held three times a day.

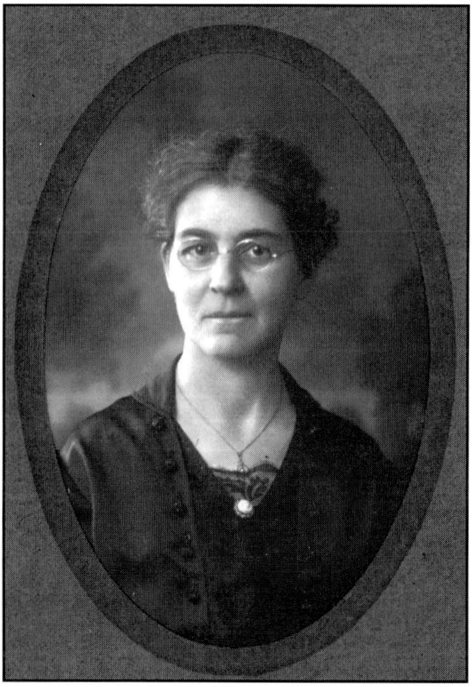

My Aunt Lala, who mortgaged her home in Greenwood to lend me money for my first year in medical school.

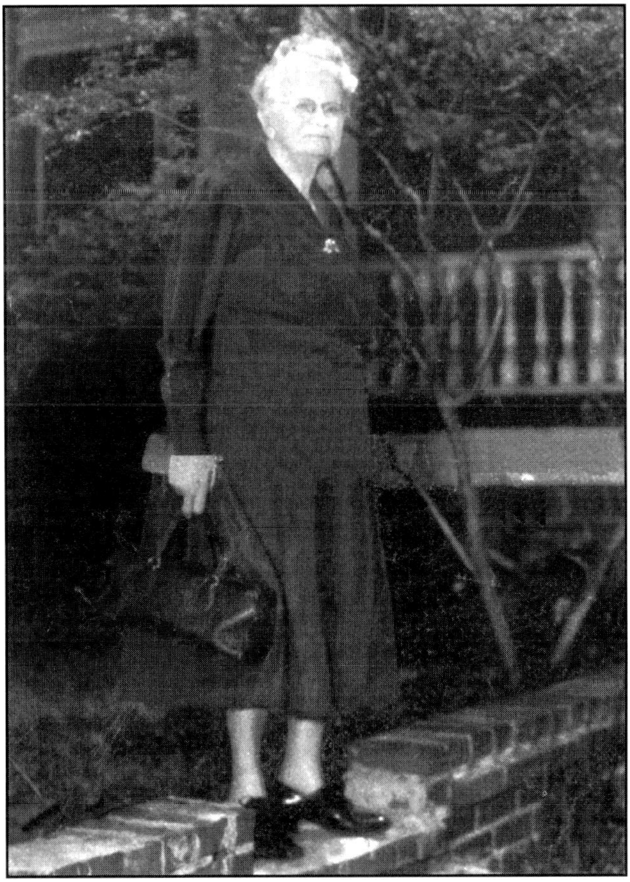

Dr. Jane Bruce Guignard, one of South Carolina's first women doctors, who lent me the money for the last three years of medical school.
– Photo courtesy of *The State* newspaper, Columbia, South Carolina

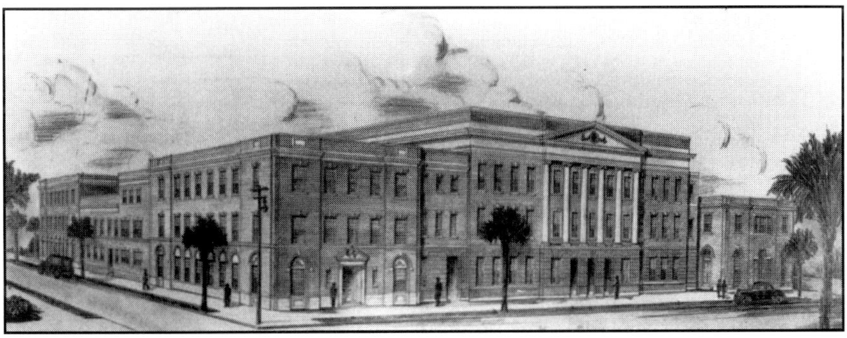

The Medical College of South Carolina circa 1943.
– Photo courtesy Archives of the Waring Historical Library, Charleston, South Carolina

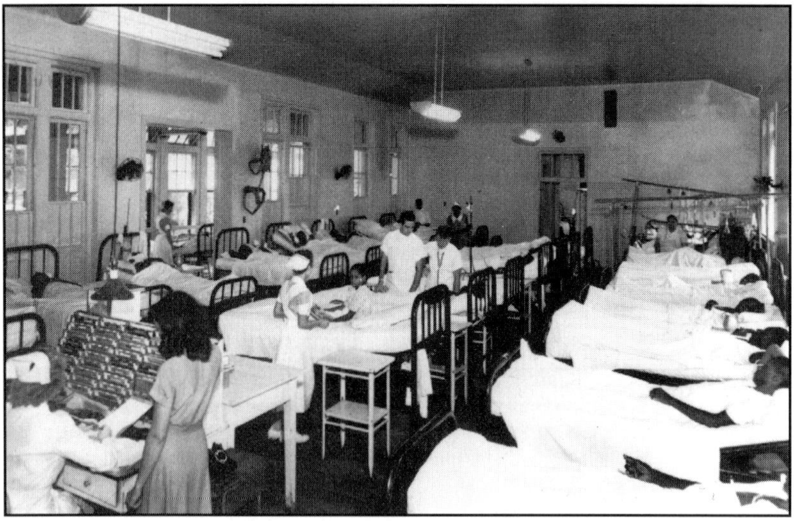

Above: *One of the wards at Roper Hospital.*
– Photo courtesy Archives of the Waring Historical Library, Charleston, South Carolina

Below:
The 1945 Pediatric Housestaff, with two faculty members, at North Carolina Baptist Hospital in Winston Salem. First row: Drs. Dan Boyette, William Venning, Jr., Robert Lawson, John Reinhart. Back row: Drs. Jefferson Beale, Jr., Martha Dukes Yow, David Schrum.

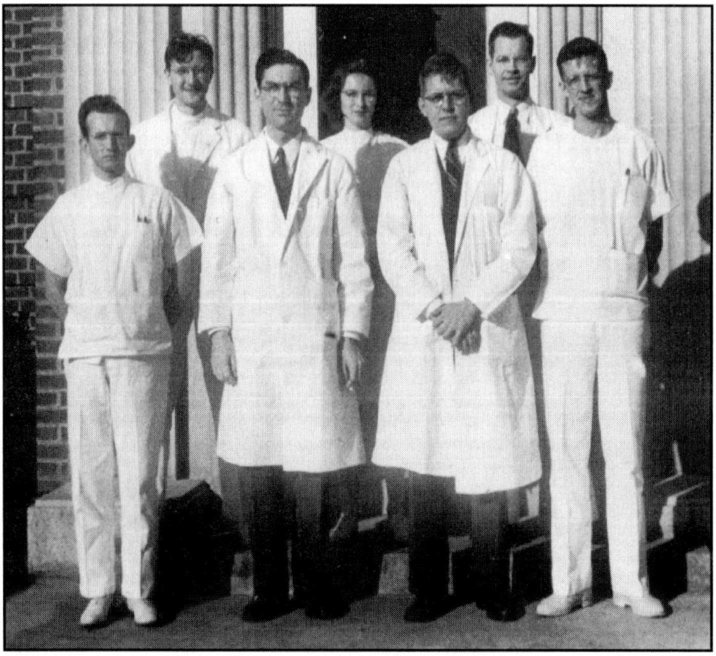

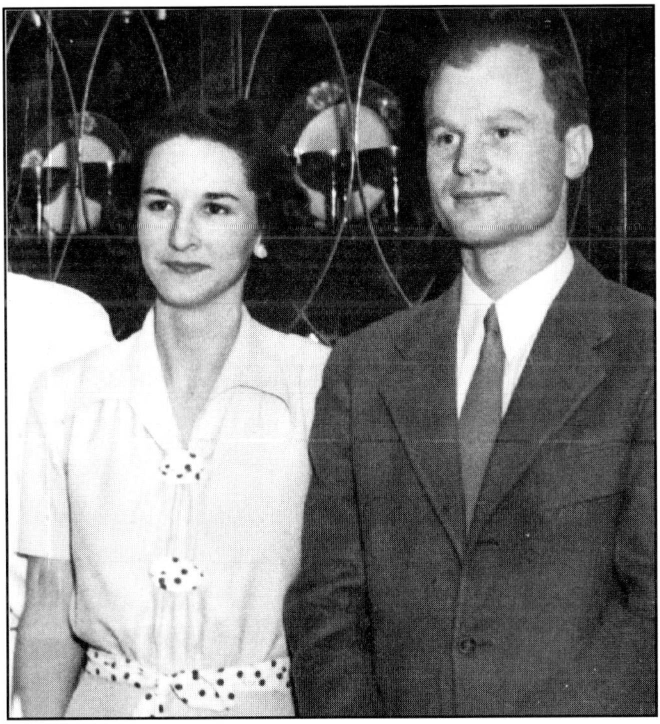

Ellard and I at our engagement party.

Below:
This is how Baylor College of Medicine looked when we arrived in 1949.

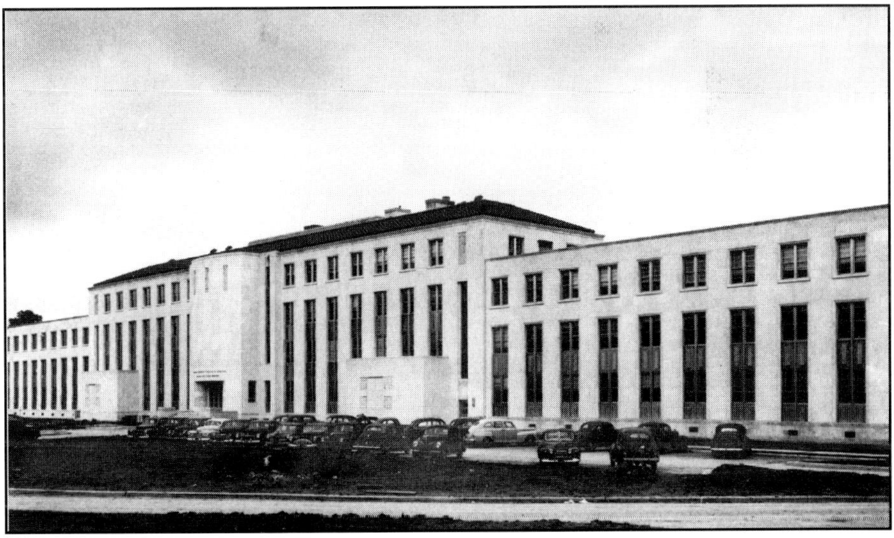

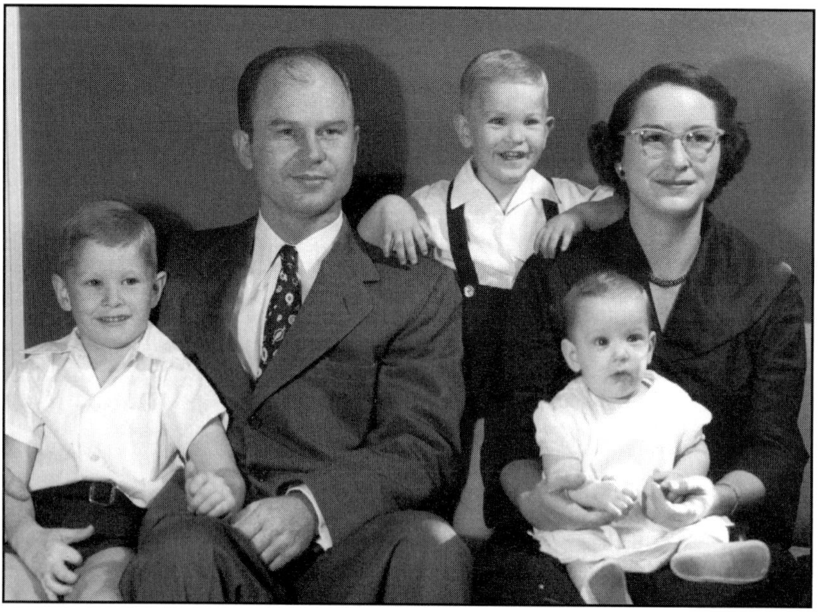

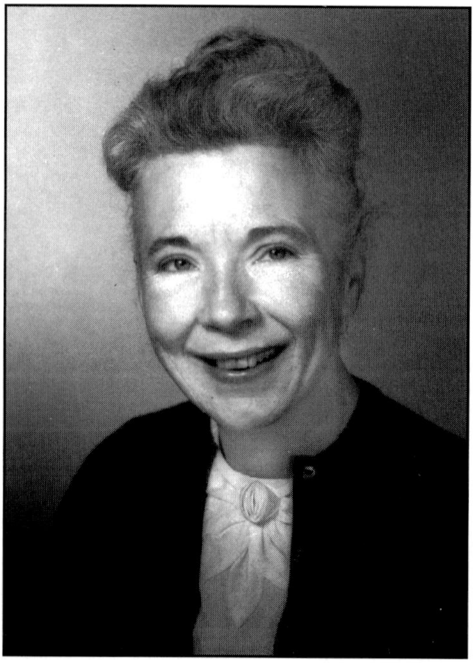

Above:
Our family in 1952 (from left to right): Ellard, Jr., Ellard, John, and Catherine sitting on my lap.

Left:
My friend, Ina Desmond, in 1958 when we were fighting the staphylococcal epidemic.

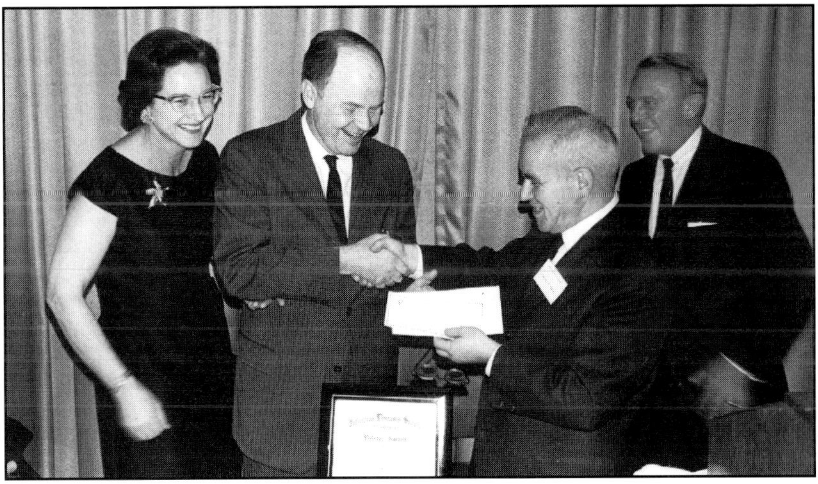

Above:
In 1964, Ellard is the recipient of the first Bristol Award of the Infectious Disease Society of America. Dr. Maxwell Finland presents the award as Dr. Charles May looks on.
Below:
Dr. Michael DeBakey talks with Catherine, Ellard, Jr., and me at the dedication of the Ellard M. Yow Memorial Library at The Methodist Hospital in Houston.

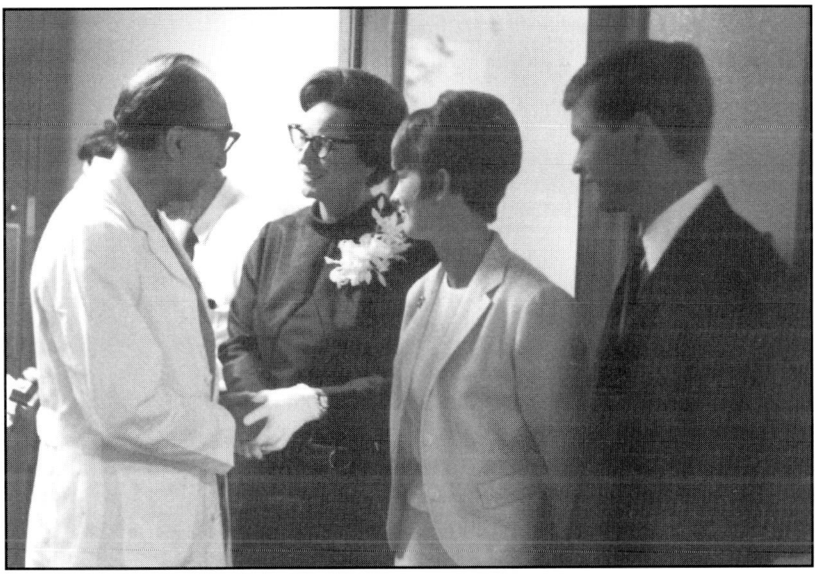

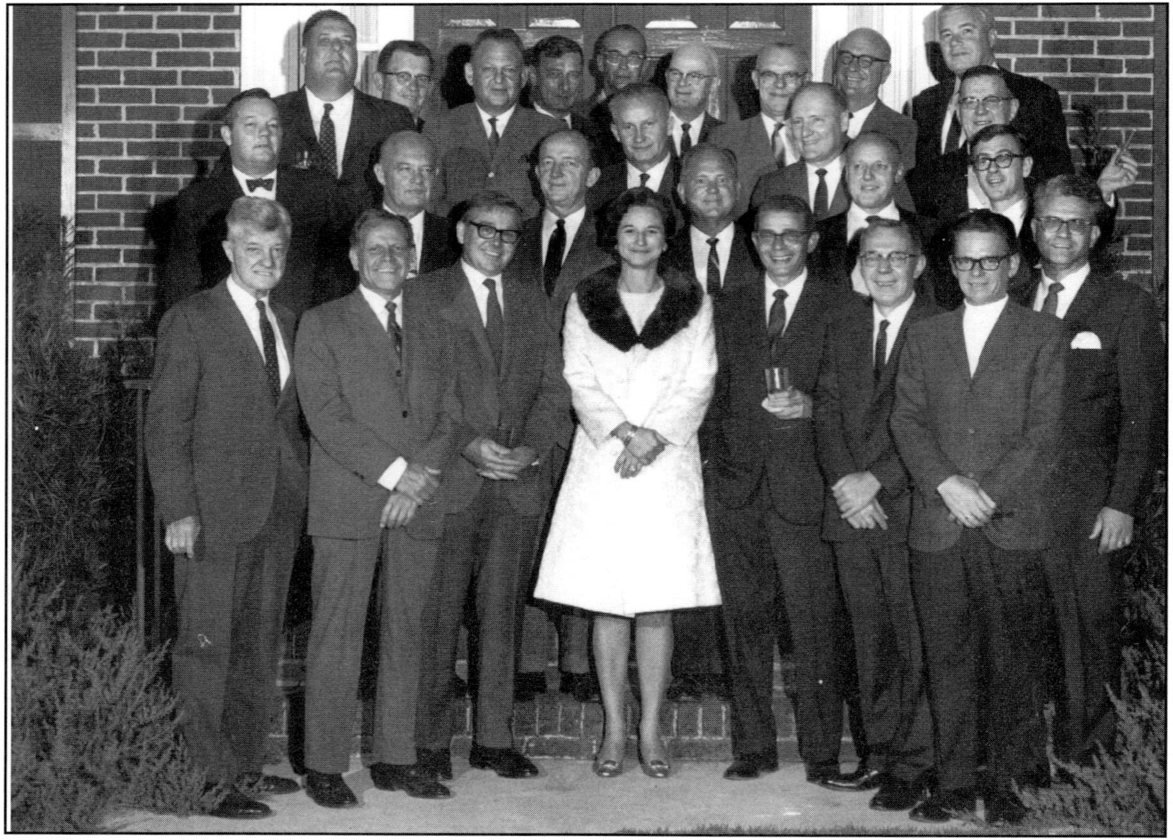

The class of December 1943 of the Medical College of South Carolina holds its 25th reunion. Front row left is one of our surgery professors, Dr. William Prioleau.

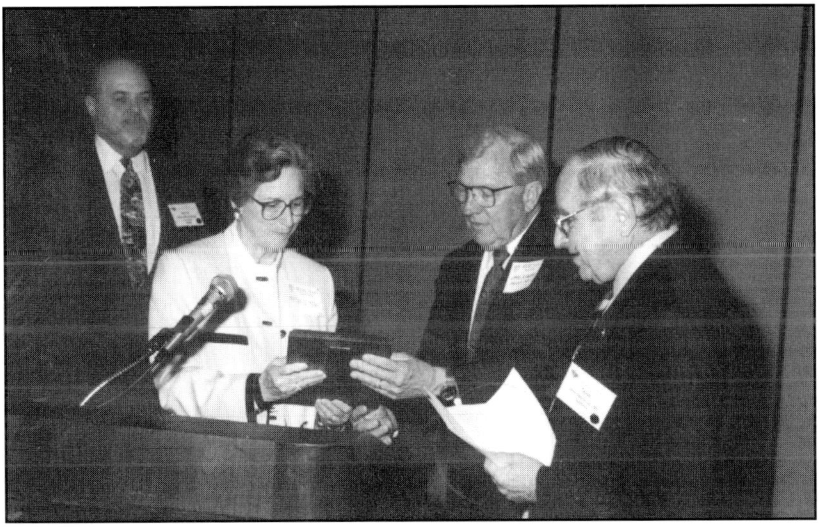

Above:

Receiving the Distinguished Alumna Award from Dr. James Edwards, President of the Medical University of South Carolina. On my left is Dr. Layton McCurdy and on Dr. Edwards' right is Dr. Leon Banov, Jr.

– Photo courtesy of the Alumni Association, Medical University of South Carolina

Left:

Good friends with me at my retirement festivities (left to right): Dr. Samuel Katz from Duke University School of Medicine, Dr. Saul Krugman from New York University School of Medicine, Dr. Marian Melish from the John A. Burns School of Medicine at the University of Hawaii, and Dr. Catherine Wilfert from Duke University School of Medicine.

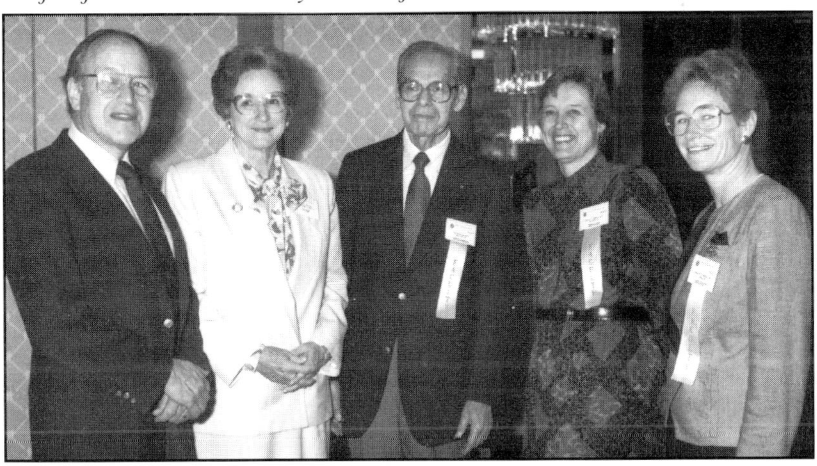

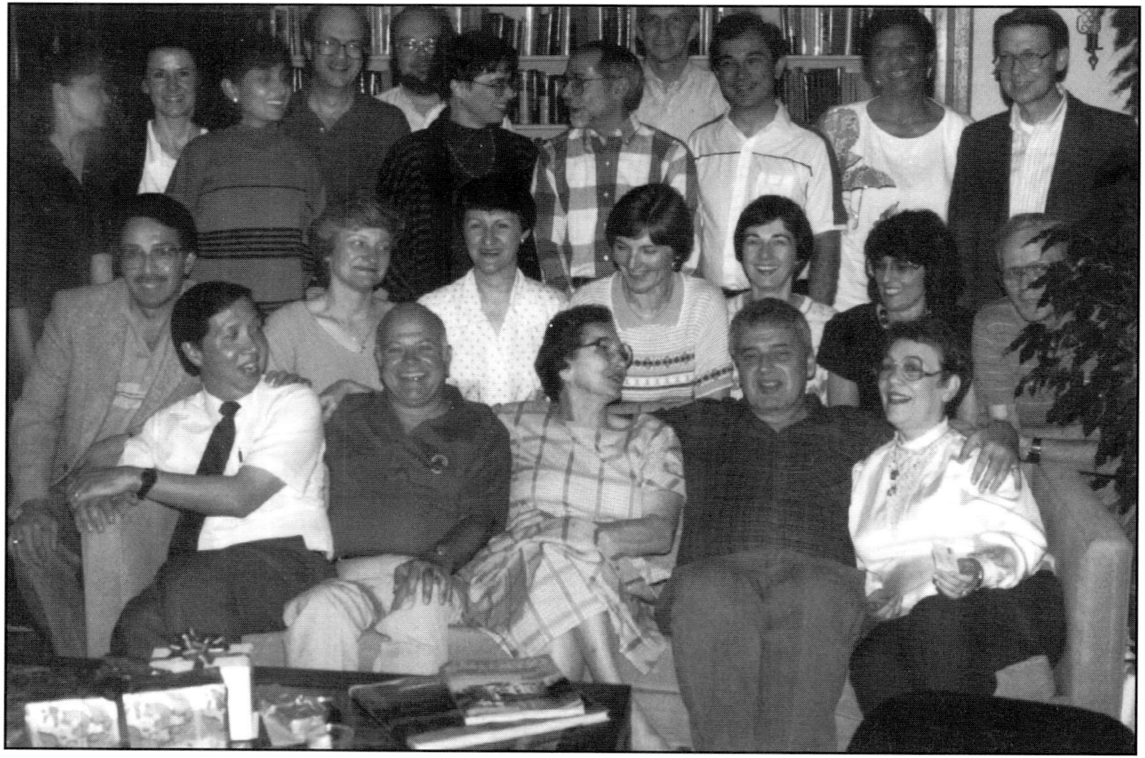

Surrounded by my fellows at our home in Houston after the formal celebration of my retirement. Front row (left to right): Drs. Peter Wong, John Montgomery, Larry Taber, and Mary Ann South.

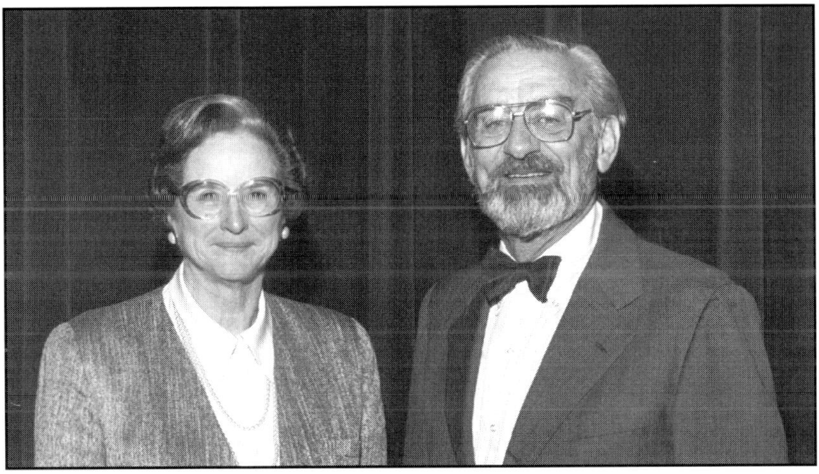

Dr. Ed Kass and I at the 1987 Annual Meeting of the Infectious Diseases Society of America held in New York. I was editor of the Journal of Infectious Diseases *and he was editor of* Reviews of Infectious Diseases. *Dr. Kass was the founder of both journals.*

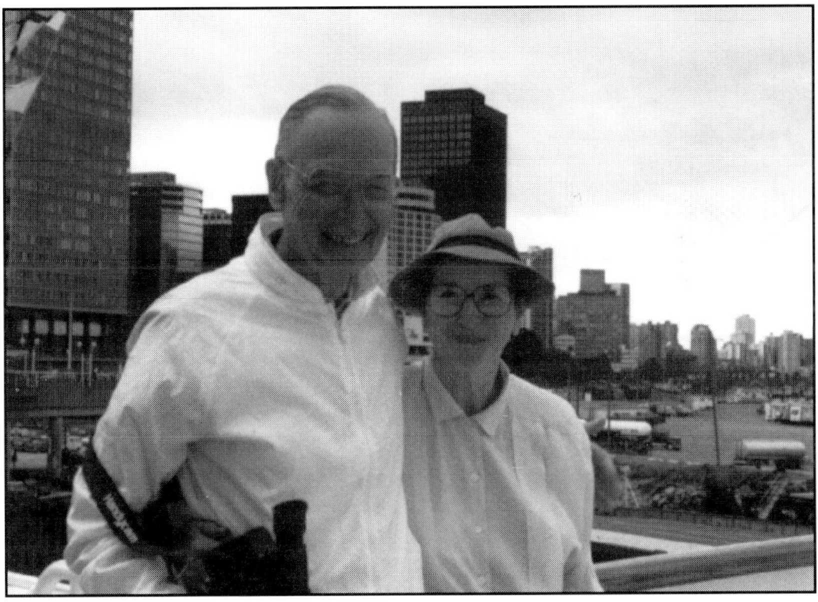

Bob and I are leaving Vancouver on an Alaskan cruise.

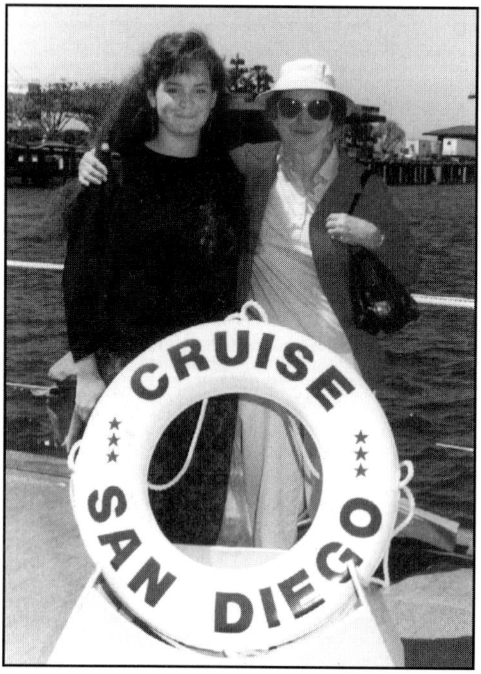

My granddaughter, Megan Keefe, and I are leaving on a harbor cruise.

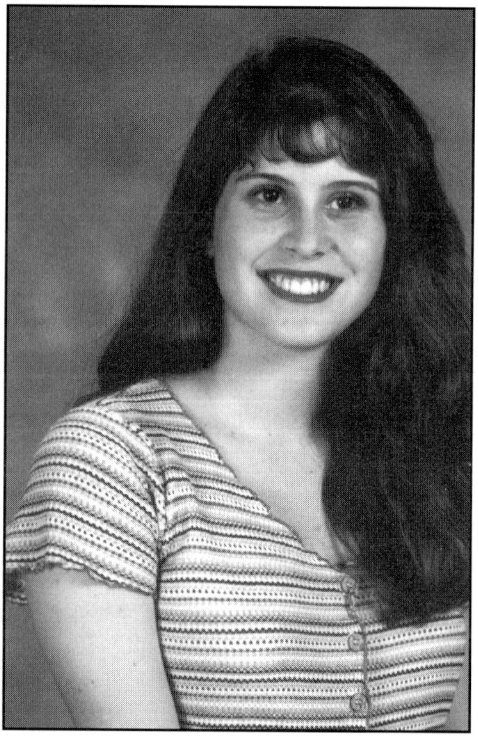

My granddaughter, Katy Yow.

infections today), but we had never tried it in children. Jack, Dr. Lawson, and I decided that, in Jimmy's case, this was the only course of action left. This seems like such a simple matter today with our modern equipment (short needles designed especially for intravenous therapy, plastic tubing that can be threaded into veins and function for days, automatic pumps for delivering fluid at a set number of drops per minute), but in 1944 it was a "do-it-yourself" undertaking.

We swung into action. Jack adapted needles for use in a child's small veins (long needles ordinarily used for intramuscular injections) by shortening them and changing the slant of the point on an emery wheel. Next we diluted the precious penicillin in a bottle of fluid, attached it to rubber tubing, and using one of Jack's needles, started a three-week course of intravenous therapy. The nurses and house officers took turns monitoring the flow of fluid every thirty minutes, day and night, by observing the level of fluid in the bottle and loosening or tightening a stopcock as necessary. Jimmy was a trooper, rarely complaining when the needle came out of the vein and had to be replaced.

Compared to similar treatment today, our methods of taking care of Jimmy were primitive, but they worked! The blood cultures became negative promptly, the fever went away in a few days, and Jimmy began to feel good. He gained weight rapidly and became an energetic little boy. When the course of penicillin was over, we kept him in the hospital for an additional two weeks, observing him for signs of relapse and performing frequent blood cultures, all of which remained free of organisms. Two and a half months after Jimmy came to the hospital, he left a happy, healthy boy, with his overjoyed parents. He was the first child that anyone on our staff had ever seen survive bacterial endocarditis.

A case that was equally gratifying was that of Bobby, a four-month-old infant with meningitis. He was brought to the hospital on a Sunday afternoon. Since early that morning he had been limp, refused to suck his bottle, and had high fever. The resident on call found that the infant's anterior fontanel (soft spot on the top of his head) was bulging from increased intracranial pressure, and knew that the most likely diagnosis was bacterial meningitis. A spinal tap was performed and, on microscopic examination, the spinal fluid was found to be loaded with pus cells. At this time, Jack Reinhart was called to see the patient. He, in turn, called me to ask me to look at the spinal fluid under the microscope and to do some special bacteriologic procedures. Jack thought that I might be able to speed up the identification of the causative organism, and needless to say, I was pleased to be considered such an expert.

I borrowed Ellard's key to Dr. Harrell's lab and sped over. Jack and I stained the spinal fluid and pored over the microscope. The specimen was loaded with pink bacteria characteristic of *Haemophilus influenzae* (*H. influenzae* – no relationship to the virus that causes influenza), the most common cause of bacterial meningitis in children. Next we used typing serum to differentiate this organism from other bacteria of similar microscopic appearance (a tedious technique not employed today). The typing proved that the bacterium was, indeed, *H. influenzae*. This finding made our hearts sink. Here was an organism that could not be eradicated by penicillin, nor could it be killed by sulfa drugs given alone. The only children who survived *H. influenzae* meningitis were those who early in their illness received an antiserum, made in rabbits, used in conjunction with a sulfa drug. This antiserum was developed by Dr. Hattie Alexander at Columbia University Medical School in New York, and she furnished the antiserum on request, only when the diagnosis was established. We had received some in the past and had administered it to children with *H. influenzae* meningitis, but we had not saved a single child. In those instances, by the time we made the diagnosis and waited for the antiserum to arrive via propeller plane, first to Atlanta and then to Winston-Salem, the illness was too far advanced for the antiserum to be effective.

On this occasion, as usual we called Dr. Alexander's laboratory to request antiserum knowing that there would be a twenty-four- to forty-eight-hour interval before we received it. But this time something was different! Dr. Harrell had been sent one gram of a new antibiotic named streptomycin. This was such a small amount that the plan was to use it for testing the susceptibility of various bacteria and perhaps to initiate treatment in one patient. The value of streptomycin was that it would kill bacteria that were not sensitive to penicillin. One gram was such a tiny amount and the drug was so highly prized that the decision concerning the manner in which it would be used was being carefully weighed. That Sunday afternoon, Jack Reinhart and I called Dr. Harrell and convinced him that our patient should be the fortunate candidate, since the one gram would be too little to treat an adult. He agreed to let us start the drug in combination with sulfadiazine. The decision to continue would depend on whether the organism proved to be sensitive to streptomycin. Now we called Ellard to join us and set up his laborious sensitivity test using a tiny amount of the precious drug. We initiated treatment of Bobby, giving him an intramuscular dose of streptomycin every three hours. Since the drug was known to penetrate poorly into the spinal fluid, we also gave him streptomycin directly into the spinal canal.

On Monday morning, Jack, Ellard and I rushed to the lab to read the sensitivity test, but it was too soon to tell whether the organism was sensitive, so we continued the streptomycin. By Tuesday the test was positive. It was clear that the *H. influenzae* organism was highly sensitive to streptomycin. Also, Bobby appeared to be improving. We had enough streptomycin to treat him for four days. Meanwhile the antiserum arrived, and the treatment was continued with it and sulfadiazine. Wonder of wonders, Bobby recovered. A short time later, two very happy residents (Jack Reinhart and Martha Yow) published this child's case report in the *North Carolina Medical Journal* (Butler, Yow & Reinhart 1946). This was the first child to recover from *H. influenzae* meningitis at North Carolina Baptist Hospital, and probably the first child in North Carolina to receive streptomycin.

The two cases of Jimmy and Bobby, along with many other cases of infectious diseases, convinced me that I loved bacteriology, being able to see the disease producing organisms under the microscope, to make a rapid and specific diagnosis, and to predict reliably what therapy might be effective. I still thought that I would practice general pediatrics, but although I reached it by a long, circuitous route, there was probably never a chance that I would end up doing anything but specializing in Pediatric Infectious Diseases.

These full, happy, stimulating days as residents passed swiftly, and in the spring of 1946, both Ellard and Jack Reinhart were called into the army since, although the war was over, the need for doctors in the service was still great. They were needed overseas to take care of the occupying forces and at home to work with the large numbers of wounded and sick servicemen being sent to military hospitals in the United States. So now I became the chief resident in Pediatrics.

Ellard was sent to Fort Knox, Kentucky, for no apparent reason, and then to Fort Sam Houston in San Antonio for basic training in the middle of the Texas summer. I received pitifully homesick letters from Ellard saying that most of the medical officers' wives were in San Antonio with them. We agreed, however, that I would stay in Winston-Salem until we knew where he would be stationed. Surprisingly, he was stationed at Brooke General Hospital at Fort Sam Houston, so five months after he left Winston-Salem, I joined him in San Antonio, four months before completing my Pediatric residency. Looking back I am amazed that neither Dr. Lawson nor the residency committee was against my leaving my residency early. Today it would be frowned upon, but the war-time climate still prevailed, and wives were expected to accompany their husbands as long as possible while they were stationed in the United States. Also there was another reason that Dr. Lawson was so understanding. Just before Ellard left, I had become pregnant and, if possible, we wanted to be together when our first child arrived. In thinking back on my days as a house officer (internship and residency), I am reminded of the advertisements for military prep schools, "Send us your boy: We'll send you back a man." That's what happened to me. I went to Winston-Salem a girl, and I left a woman.

Chapter 7

The Pediatrician Learns About Babies

THE MOVE TO TEXAS marked a major transition in my life. For the first time in almost a decade, my drive was not toward being a doctor. Now I was immersed in becoming a mother and in finding an adequate place to live. My arrival in San Antonio was something of a shock. Ellard had written that San Antonio was like Florida with lots of beautiful palm trees and that when I arrived, we would stay at the elegant, Spanish-style officer's club for a few days while we looked for an apartment. After the intense work of being a house officer, I looked forward to lolling around the club pool surrounded by palm trees rustling in the breeze. It was not to be. As we rode away from the airport, Ellard explained to me that we would not be going to the officers' club, but to a hotel where we would live for a while in order to get in line for one of the tourist cabins adjacent to the hotel. He said that several of his fellow officers and their wives were there also waiting in line.

Nothing had prepared me for El Grande Hotel, a two-story, weathered, frame building next to a small tortilla factory on the edge of the barrio. There was not a palm tree in sight. And nothing had prepared me for the blast furnace heat of a Texas September. I felt sure that having grown up in low country South

Carolina, heat would never really bother me, but I was mistaken. I hadn't experienced Texas heat. Many San Antonio homes and buildings were built with thick walls, terra cotta roofs, and wide overhanging eaves. The El Grande Hotel was not one of them, but it did provide shade, and I learned to stay indoors as much as possible. Each morning after Ellard left for the army post, I waited to see whether some couple was moving out of a cabin in El Grande Courts, so that our name could inch up on the list. I was also spending a great deal of time at the pay phone in the lobby answering ads about apartments. It was to no avail. Either the apartments were far beyond a lieutenant's price range, their locations weren't on a bus line, or the landlord would not accept children. I tried to avoid the landlord's inevitable question, "Are you pregnant?" but when I had to answer, "Yes," I hastened to explain that I was only five months pregnant, and that the baby wouldn't be out of the crib for months, so it couldn't damage anything. That fell on deaf ears – no children!

At the hotel, I met other wives who were in the same predicament, and we walked around ringing doorbells asking for housing. It was not rewarding. San Antonio was flooded with soldiers and their wives, and there was no housing on the post for married men below the rank of major. So we all spent our two weeks or so of purgatory in the El Grande Hotel and then we moved into one of the standard twelve foot square cabins of El Grande Courts.

The front door opened directly off a narrow side walk into a bedroom furnished with an iron bedstead, a rocking chair and a straight chair. The area across the back of the cabin was divided into a tiny kitchen, a dining area, and a minuscule bathroom. The bedroom had four windows one on each side and two on either side of the front door. Bedraggled net curtain panels hung over the windows. The back door led to a small space equipped with clotheslines and the cabins were about three feet apart, so it was truly communal living. We could hear everything said by the people in the cabins on either side of us, and they, in turn, heard everything we said. Visual privacy was provided by the stringy curtains.

Despite the obvious limitations of the cabin, Ellard and I were thrilled to move from the hotel; we could at least cook for ourselves. This was the first time we had been able to eat at home since we were married. I had never cooked a meal in those first three years. I'll never forget the impassioned blessing Ellard said at the first meal I cooked in El Grande Courts, "Thank you, God, for this wonderful food and for my wonderful wife!"

Also we were convinced that by January, when the baby was due, we would find a real apartment, after all this was only September and we had ample opportunity to improve our circumstances. We were dreaming. We were to live in El Grande Courts for six months.

The time from September to January was pleasant. There were several other couples from Winston Salem living in El Grande Courts and we had lots in common. All the husbands were stationed at Brooke General Hospital and all the wives were pregnant. We wives enjoyed each other and we caught the bus and went downtown shopping for maternity clothes and layettes. The other wives showed me how to make receiving blankets and other mysterious layette items. We made bassinets out of laundry baskets, though mine looked like something a six-year-old child had decorated. Once a week, we caught the bus and went to the commissary to grocery shop. Ellard and I allotted forty dollars a month for groceries and managed quite well by eating lots of peanut butter and tuna fish.

On the weekends, the couples played cards at our tiny dinette tables. If anybody had to go to the bathroom, everybody had to stand up and push the table to one side so that the bathroom door could be opened. I had a pretty active social life, because Ellard and I studied the protocol followed by regular army officers and made formal calls on his superior officers and their wives. Two of these wives adopted me and incorporated me into their weekly bridge game. This meant they had to pick me up at El Grande Courts and transport me to their lovely Spanish homes on the post. Although my bridge was not very good, it was a glorious treat.

These were easy days for me. I was not apprehensive about having the baby or taking care of it. I would have caudal anaesthesia, an injection at the very end of the spinal cord, so the delivery would be a snap; and after all, I was a pediatrician and knew all about babies! What was there to be concerned about?

Around the first of December, Ellard came home very excited. He reported that we had a great stroke of luck. A medical officer who was going overseas had a car he wanted to sell. During the immediate post war years, buying a car was almost impossible unless one had a car to trade in. So we bought an eleven-year-old Air Flow DeSoto for three hundred dollars. We knew that it was held together with bailing wire, had retreaded tires and dim, non-sealed beam headlights. There was obviously a hole in the muffler because the motor roared loudly, but we didn't mind – we had transportation. Soon, Ellard had to repair some part of the car almost every day, using adhesive tape, tongue depressors, and surgical wire. He depleted my layette by taking a Kleinert baby pad to stop a leak in the roof. Now Ellard and his colleagues could ride directly to the post instead of taking the bus downtown and transferring to another bus. Each morning except Wednesday, they roared off in splendor. On Wednesday, I got to keep the car so that the wives had transportation for grocery shopping; a great help, since with our ever increasing girths, carrying groceries on the bus became more and more difficult.

The great day arrived. On January 13th I called Ellard at the post to say that I was having labor pains. There was no urgency, but in his excitement, he rushed home where he kept me active every minute. He didn't want the labor to stop! First I had to help install fog screens on the windshield of the car (San Antonio had heavy morning fog in the winter). Then he had me walking up and down the hilly streets around El Grande Courts. Finally about seven that night my contractions were frequent enough that we went to the hospital. This was before the days of husband participation during labor and delivery, so he kissed me goodbye and I was wheeled into the labor room. By then I was having severe pains, so the doctor started the caudal anaesthesia, and a "caudal nurse" was assigned to me. The caudal anaesthesia worked beautifully and I felt no pain during contractions. The resident on call that night turned out to be none other than my woman classmate from medical school. She and I talked and talked, told stories and laughed. Apparently the nurse wanted me to go to sleep, and despite my protestations that I was having no pain, she gave me several doses of demerol. After the first, I was so dopey that I didn't protest much about the other doses, but the amount of demerol that I received in one night was certainly excessive, and it must have slowed or stopped my labor, because at 7:00 A.M. the doctor came and told me that he had spent the night in the hospital thinking that I would deliver. He listened to the fetal heart tones and appeared concerned. In 1947 there were no mechanical monitoring devices. One listened through the mother's abdominal wall using a special stethoscope. He was not happy about what he heard and quickly ruptured the membranes to stimulate labor. Within two hours I had a beautiful, red-haired boy, Ellard, Jr.

Ellard, Sr., turned into an ecstatic and vocal father. I, in turn, became the penultimate mother. Breast feeding was not in vogue, but I was determined to breast feed because I knew the nutritional and immunologic advantages. I tried and I cried. Ellard, Jr. arrived in my hospital room crying and left crying. He sucked and sucked, but I had tender, engorged breasts and the breast feeding seemed not to satisfy him, so the nurses gave him a supplemental formula. They gave me a hand breast pump to use, but offered no instruction or assistance. The wonderful electric breast pump was not yet available, and since breast feeding was not especially promoted, there was no emphasis on helping mothers to do so. I asked the nurses whether the baby cried a lot in the nursery since he was always crying when I saw him. They assured me that he slept like a lamb. I didn't visit him in the nursery, because new mothers were kept virtually in bed or sitting up for about a week. My hospital stay lasted the customary week, and then the baby and I went home to El Grande Courts where I was sure I could manage perfectly.

What a rude awakening, and awakening is the right word. It seemed that we were never to sleep again. The beautiful baby cried and cried. He seemed insatiable. He breast fed, then took supplemental formula until his little abdomen was as tight as a drum, and still he wanted to suck. Pacifiers were a no-no but we tried to make him one by filling a bottle nipple with cotton. He was so young that he couldn't keep it in his mouth. Finally, at night we got so desperate that we washed our hands thoroughly with soap, alcohol, and then clear water, put the baby between us and alternated letting him suck our fingers. When the sucker went to sleep and the finger fell out of his mouth, he would scream and then it became the other parent's turn.

When young Ellard was three weeks old, he weighed less than his birth weight which really alarmed us. The degree of his father's concern was evident one night when he was taking his shift walking the baby, and I was supposed to be sleeping. This particular night, the sounds of Ellard's steps were step, step, slide (the rocking chair being pushed out of the way), step, step, slide, and in his crooning, he said, "Poor little baby. We'll never raise you." With that I burst into loud sobs. Ellard was so exhausted that he yelled, "You're supposed to be sleeping. If you're not going to sleep, get up and walk this baby!"

At this point, our pediatrician pronounced the baby "colicky" and felt that my breast milk might be causing the trouble, so he recommended that I discontinue breast feeding. Regrettably, I did. Then came the usual series of formula changes, none of which helped. Finally we settled on one that we thought might have some advantages, but the crying and poor sleeping continued. We would not have been quite so worried if the baby had been gaining weight. We felt that he didn't have simple colic, because infants with colic usually gain normally. We never found out the reason for young Ellard's excessive crying and sucking, although I always suspected that the large doses of demerol I received during labor and the interruption of labor had something to do with it. In any event, to our great relief, at about a month of age, he gradually began to gain weight.

The sleeping, however, improved very little, because Ellard, Jr. was extremely jittery. The least little noise startled him so I learned to perform any noisy cooking tasks out behind the cabin. His formula was difficult to dissolve in water and required vigorous mixing with an egg beater. This was carried out under the clotheslines. Dishes had to be washed quietly. We moved about in our tiny space tiptoeing and whispering. Fortunately we had no phone to ring.

Ellard, Jr. slept little in the daytime and virtually none at night. I remember holding him and crying as I read the pediatric book that described the newborn infant's sleeping pattern as being sixteen to twenty hours per twenty-four hours.Why didn't the pediatric text explain what to do about sleeping problems? Why hadn't I learned anything about them during my training? We tried everything; we held him, we rocked him, we walked him. Our pediatrician friends came by and insisted they could get him to sleep, but they went home defeated. He seemed to need to be held close, and I suspect old fashioned swaddling would have helped him. That, too, was out of style, so we never even considered it. Usually he fell asleep about 6:00 A.M., and Ellard, Sr. crept around dressing as quietly as possible. Then he would kiss me goodby and whisper, "you're going to have a good day." He slipped out the front door, but at the first roar of the car just outside the door, a few feet from the bassinet, Ellard, Jr. leapt to attention and the day had begun.

As I mentioned, breast feeding, swaddling, and pacifiers were not in vogue, but mother-bashing definitely was. If a baby was tense, it was always ascribed to the mother's being tense; never the other way around. If the infant did not thrive on breast milk, it was because the milk was too weak or the mother was too nervous. It makes me sad to remember those difficult days, but many parents in my later practice benefitted from my experiences. I never again automatically assumed that if a baby was having trouble, the mother was doing something wrong. I learned two valuable lessons; that nobody knows a child as well as his parents, and that it is important to listen to parents. Every pediatrician should have to deal with a child who is jittery, a child who can't sleep, and one who has colic. Some pediatricians do not even believe that colic is an entity. I can assure them that it is real.

We lived like this for two months during which Ellard, Jr. slowly began to gain weight, while both of his parents lost weight. The baby never slept for any prolonged time until we had the great and wonderful fortune to move into a converted army barracks where we could move about without disturbing him. Then we all began to relax. We were still up about 5:00 A.M. each day, but things were infinitely better. We had weathered the first two months of a new baby's life. The colicky period was over, and he had his days and nights straightened out.

Before we left El Grande Courts where I was crying every day and thinking, "I can't look at these four walls and eight stringy curtains another day," I got a call from a woman pediatrician in San Antonio. She, too, was having a baby and wanted to know whether I would run her practice for about six months. I told her no, that there was no way I could work and leave our baby. That night when I laughingly told Ellard about her call, he caught me completely off guard by saying, "I think you ought to do it. You're shut in here and crying all the time. I think you should get a nurse for the baby and try working. We'll be moving into the barracks soon and will have room for a daytime nurse."

I couldn't believe my ears. How could anybody take care of my precious baby as well as I could? Only I knew how he liked to be held and how he liked to be fed! But despite conflicting feelings, I called the pediatrician to tell her I would work for her for a short time. Little did I realize that I was beginning a life-long balancing act between my need or wish to work as a doctor and my desire to be a perfect wife and mother.

* * * * * * * *

The opportunity to serve a *locum tenens*, the temporary management of another doctor's practice, was a real break for me. There was no teaching hospital in San Antonio where I could continue my training, and, of course, I didn't consider going into practice, because at most, we would be in San Antonio two years. In fact it was impossible to make any long-term plans because we had no idea how long Ellard would be assigned to Brooke General Hospital. As it turned out, he spent two years there, and I worked as a substitute general pediatrician for a year and a half. I was fortunate to have all the arrangements made for me. I knew absolutely nothing about organizing and financing an office and here I was with an established practice, a well-equipped office, a good nurse, and an outstanding receptionist-office manager. The latter had been a sergeant in the army and she knew how to run that office!

I needed all the help I could get. I was young (twenty-five) and green. My training in a hospital with seriously ill children had not prepared me for office practice. Now I was seeing many normal newborns and counseling their mothers, providing well baby care, learning about growth and development, and treating common childhood diseases, such as sore throats, infected ears, skin problems, and minor injuries. I made lots of mistakes and would have made more, had the nurse not guided me. I had special problems diagnosing skin rashes. I misdiagnosed infected chigger bites as chickenpox, and wondered why the patient's siblings didn't catch it. Numerous home remedies were prescribed by Mexican-American grandmothers to "flush the poisons out" of the niños, and some of these herbal teas caused bright red rashes that I thought were roseola or three-day measles until the nurse diplomatically asked the mother whether the baby had received one of these ritual concoctions.

My most ignominious experience in diagnosing a skin problem occurred when I saw an infant with an unusual rash that I thought might be due to congenital syphilis. Of course, I did not discuss this suspicion with the mother. I drew a blood sample for "tests" and in this particular instance, I had a great deal of difficulty obtaining the blood and having to bend down closely over the baby with him crying into my face. In a few days I received a negative report for syphilis and since the rash was fading and the infant was improving, I ordered no further diagnostic procedures, thinking I would probably never know the cause of the rash. Two weeks later, however, I knew the diagnosis. I, myself, had a rip-roaring case of German measles (three-day measles).

Not only did I learn about common childhood problems, I also learned about the difficulties of private practice and the constancy of it. I was handling a solo practice and the demands seemed unending; office hours five and a half days a week and available the rest of the time. Occasionally I signed out to another pediatrician, but most of the time I was on call. Answering services were not routine and the beeper had not come into existence, so nights and weekends my home phone rang constantly, especially during the dinner hour. Characteristically children have the highest fever in late afternoon and early evening. This resulted not only in disruption of our home life, but often necessitated night time house calls. In the 1940s, patients were not sent to emergency rooms unless it was a real emergency. They were seen in their homes by their private doctors.

I probably made more house calls than necessary, because of inexperience. It takes time to develop judgment as to which situation demands an immediate examination and which can be handled by telephone, and it also requires knowledge of your clientele. After a period of working with parents, one gets to know which parents call about the slightest problem and simply need reassurance, and which ones call only when problems are urgent. In my situation, I didn't know the parents well enough to take any chances, so I made lots of house calls.

Although I appreciated the pediatric experience I was gaining, as well as the opportunity to begin to repay my medical school debts, my working put a severe strain on our marriage. For the first time we were experiencing the difficulties associated with both parents working outside of the home. Our situation was no longer that of two friends working side by side with no major home duties. Now each of us had a demanding, responsible, time-consuming job, and when we came home, there was supper to prepare, a baby to take care of, and a telephone that never seemed to stop ringing.

We handled the situation poorly. We were of a generation that assumed that the man made the living and when he came home he was not responsible for cooking or child care. If the woman worked outside the home, she was solely responsible for child care, marketing, cooking, and all other domestic chores. We had a combination housekeeper-baby nurse five and a half days a week, but there was no overlap in our schedules. When I got home, she left. That meant that I had no leisure time at all.

Ellard and I should have known better, but we didn't. I felt resentful and overtaxed and Ellard felt that he had a tired, irritable wife with little enthusiasm for social life. In addition, the car kept breaking down, so Ellard had to spend much of his spare time assuring our transportation. Several times he came in after a grueling session with the car's rusted parts and said, "I'm going to drive the damned thing in the ditch and leave it!"

Surprisingly, I agreed with Ellard that I should take care of all the domestic duties. I had thoroughly absorbed the attitude of society and felt that I should be submissive and do whatever Ellard wanted me to do. I had gotten the impression that my mother's working outside the home and being the leader of the family had contributed to my parents' marital troubles. As a child, I had been so heart broken over the dysfunction and eventual dissolution of our family, that I was determined to have a good marriage and a good home regardless of the adaptations I had to make. Also growing up in the south, I had gotten a confused idea of the ideal woman. I thought to be a good wife, one had to assume a sweet, subordinate role, and it was a number of years before I understood the myth of the soft, adoring little Southern wife and replaced it with the more realistic knowledge that, although some women were genuinely gentle and loving, others hid the iron fist in the velvet glove. I came to realize that women with the most gentle facades were often the most manipulative and controlling. Needless to say, my ignorance about appropriate degrees of dependence between spouses and my strong need for Ellard's approval were bad for both of us.

Today's young couples have different expectations and less rigid role definitions, and discuss the sharing of home responsibilities. However, I suspect that in many instances the sharing works less well than is reported. Certainly, surveys show that working wives in the 1990s are still performing the lion's share of the domestic duties.

The pervasive attitude about the lack of importance of a woman's career was evident when Ellard began planning what to do after his army service. We briefly discussed his going into practice in North Carolina, but he decided that he wanted to pursue a career in academic medicine. This required further training, and he decided to use his money from the G.I. bill to take a fellowship in infectious diseases at The University of Minnesota. It never occurred to either of us that I should have the same opportunity. We just assumed that I would go along and run the home. Today when one member of a medical couple is recruited, the recruiting institution makes every effort to give the spouse a position, but at that time, trying to get two appointments in the same place was so far from the normal procedure that we didn't even consider it.

* * * * * * * *

In April 1948, we headed north with our fifteen-month-old son to live in graduate school quarters at the University in Minneapolis. This time there was to be no house hunting. The

University had made the arrangements, and we were assigned to one half of a quonset hut. The half was a single twelve by twenty foot room with no partitions except for one tiny corner which contained a toilet. There was no basin, no shower, no tub. The far end of the room next to the bathroom door had a stove, an icebox, a kitchen counter, and a sink. All hand washing and bathing had to be done at the kitchen sink. For a real bath or shower, one went out of doors to a central shower room in the midst of the quonsets. We bathed young Ellard in the sink, and we went to the shower room. This didn't seem too bad in April, but we shuddered to think of going out for a bath in Minnesota's sub-zero weather. There were other drawbacks, such as no outside play area for children . . . just patchy areas of dirty snow covered with cinders to prevent falls.

Many graduate students with wives and several children were living in these slum-like conditions, but Ellard said that an education wasn't worth it and vowed that if we couldn't improve the situation, I should take Ellard, Jr. and go back to North Carolina or South Carolina while he was in training. We didn't come to that pass, though, because soon we found a "winterized" cottage on Cedar Lake on the opposite side of town from the University and were thrilled.

It was spring and people were bursting out of their houses to enjoy the warmer weather. We made friends quickly and our neighbors enjoyed the naive Southern newcomers, especially when they donned bathing suits and jumped in the lake about the middle of May. They watched from their porches as we made a rapid entry and an even more rapid exit. Later we were informed that the ice had been out of the lake only two weeks when we took our initial plunge. Not to be outdone, though, we continued to swim daily. Being on the lake was a wonderful thing for our energetic little boy who still had sleeping problems. I took him swimming before lunch and let him wear himself out. He could hardly stay awake to have his lunch and then he took a nap. Before supper, either his father or I took him for another swim, and after eating he could usually go to sleep for the night. If not, his Dad took him for a third swim. Young Ellard learned to swim before he could talk, and he learned to sleep!

After we were settled in our pleasant home, I investigated

the possibility of continuing my education at the University Hospital. I hoped to complete my pediatric residency, but there was no Pediatric residency available at the hospital. Doctors returning from military duty were clamoring for training and residency programs everywhere were full. However, I was offered a research fellowship investigating the possible role of respiratory viruses in the sudden infant death syndrome. It looked interesting, but I would have to be on call day and night to collect specimens and to assist in autopsies. I knew that arrangement would jeopardize my marriage so I turned down the opportunity. I gave up the idea of working during the year we would be in Minneapolis, but fate intervened. One day in the fall, a woman pediatrician invited me to accompany her to a one-day pediatric seminar in Eau Claire, Wisconsin. At the seminar I met a Minneapolis pediatrician, who asked me whether I was doing any medical work. When I replied that I was not, he asked whether I would be interested in working part-time. I told him I would have to think it over and discuss it with my husband. That night when I told Ellard about the offer, his bad feelings about my San Antonio work surfaced. He said, "I don't mind if you work if I can't tell you're working." I felt that his comment was unfair, but I decided to give the job a try.

I found a college girl who could come to our home each weekday by 1:00 P.M., so in the mornings I cleaned house, took Ellard out to play, and fed him before I left him with her. Then I caught the bus, bundled up against the wind blowing across the lake, and went down town to work until six. When I got home, I had to fix supper before making any house calls assigned to me. House calls were especially hard, because I was unfamiliar with the city and often street signs were plastered with snow and unreadable. One night after searching and searching and wading across a wide field of snow, I arrived at a home where a little girl had a fiery strep throat and needed a shot of penicillin (oral penicillins had not yet been developed). When I reached in my black bag for the alcohol to cleanse her skin, the bottle was empty. I thought about the long way back to get alcohol and quickly dismissed the idea. I asked the father, "Do you have any whiskey?" He produced a bottle of bourbon and I washed the skin with soap and water, gave it a generous swabbing with Jack Daniel's and administered the penicillin.

While I was in Minnesota I got my first introduction to efficiently administered well-baby care to relatively poor children. One day a month, I kept the car and drove thirty miles out of town along Lake Minnetonka to a school where I saw about thirty babies in an afternoon. The system was unlike anything I had ever seen. It functioned like a smoothly running belt-line assembly. A Junior League volunteer recorded the pertinent history, the baby was then placed on the table in front of me, and I examined his eyes, ears, nose, throat, heart, lungs, abdomen, genitalia, and extremities. An assistant flipped him over like a pancake, and I examined his back and hips. Next the infant passed on by to the next table where a nurse gave him the scheduled immunization. Then he was dressed and gone. There was little conversation, and when I ventured a few questions or pleasantries, the Minnesota housewives looked askance; the young southern doctor seemed to want to be too friendly. On those afternoons, I was paid fifteen dollars for examining thirty infants. But the money didn't matter. I was seeing my first good preventive medicine and I got to ride along Lake Minnetonka in the glory of all four seasons.

We enjoyed our time in Minnesota – the lovely summer, the adventure of living in the snowy winter. I even managed to shed some of my provincialism and realized that people north of the Mason Dixon Line could be wonderful neighbors and friends. We would have stayed in Minnesota longer, but Ellard had been offered a job at Baylor College of Medicine, the new school in Houston, Texas, and when he asked whether he could spend another year in fellowship at the University of Minnesota, he was told that he was needed at Baylor and that it was "now or never."

Chapter 8

Homesteading in Texas

NINETEEN FORTY-NINE WAS A wonderful time to move to Houston! It was a booming vibrant city with a small-town feel. The city had not yet become hermetically sealed, by air conditioning, and Houstonians still sat on porches and had backyard picnics, despite the intense heat and humidity. There was a delightful air of hospitality and openness, and in the summer, there was a certain amount of enforced leisure, if only to stay cool. The great exodus to the suburbs had not begun and downtown was still a wonderful place to shop. People were moving to Houston from all over the world because of the oil industry, the busy seaport, and the new medical center, creating an interesting mix of hearty native Texans and newcomers.

When Ellard and I arrived in Houston, we thought our move to Baylor University College of Medicine was the first of perhaps several moves during his academic career, since doctors in academic medicine usually advanced up the ladder by changing medical schools at intervals. Many people questioned the wisdom of our move to Houston and Baylor. Our academic colleagues in Minnesota felt that Ellard should go to a more established medical center, such as Harvard or Hopkins, and they openly voiced the opinion that there was no medical opportunity in Houston, exclaiming, "There is nothing there!" Their attitude seems especially funny as I write this in the 1990s, when the Texas Medical Center in Houston is one of the largest and finest medical centers in the world. Members of our families had different reasons for wondering about what we were doing. First, they questioned why Ellard had chosen academic medicine instead of a nice, remunerative private practice, and why, if he wanted to do academic medicine had he chosen Texas instead of the Southeast. I was still making no active plans about my medical career, but I understood Ellard's attraction to academic medicine.

When Ellard was offered a position as an assistant professor at Baylor, we knew it was the perfect choice. The school was in a period of expansion, so that Ellard could participate in its development instead of being merely "a cog in the machine" in an established school. And it was near the sea, too!

Baylor was not really a new school, but it had been moved from Dallas to Houston just about three years before we arrived in 1949. Philanthropists in Houston had made prime land and money available for the move and development of the school there. Although some of the Dallas faculty moved with the school, there was also vigorous recruitment of new faculty, including the Chairman of the Department of Medicine, Dr. James Green, from the University of Iowa Medical School; the chairman of the Department of Surgery, Dr. Michael DeBakey, from Tulane University in New Orleans, and the chairman of Pediatrics, Dr. Russell Blattner, from Washington University in St. Louis.

We arrived at exactly just the right time. The school had originally been housed in an old Sears warehouse, but had recently moved into its new location in The Texas Medical Center. It was an attractive four-story white limestone building set in the middle of a pine forest, one of only two structures in the medical center; the other was Hermann Hospital. (Today the pine trees are long gone and the Texas Medical Center is a vast complex of two medical schools and many hospitals and institutions.) From Baylor, the hospital was reached by crossing a wooden foot bridge over a small stream. Hermann was originally to have been the teaching hospital for Baylor; the two institutions were ideally situated for this association, but some sort of political upheaval occurred, and to our dismay, by the time we arrived, the agreement no longer existed. Jefferson Davis Hospital, the large city-county hospital, twenty minutes from the medical school through heavy traffic, had become the teaching hospital.

Jefferson Davis Hospital (J.D., as it was called) was a typical big city charity hospital of that era. It was horribly overcrowded, dirty, underfinanced, unairconditioned, and there was virtually no office space. The enthusiastic young Baylor faculty made the arduous trip, in hot, unairconditioned cars back and forth to J.D. daily, and frequently more than once.

Somehow Ellard obtained a small room that he made into a lab in order to offer the best possible care to the patients with infectious diseases. Here he began to test the sensitivity of patients' organisms to a new type of antibiotic, tetracycline, and used it to treat infections for which previously there had been no treatment. He had been working with this antibiotic in Minnesota and the pharmaceutical firm that produced it gave him $5,000 worth of this drug to bring to Baylor. Occasionally when our budget at home was particularly tight he would jokingly say, "I think I should sell the tetracycline. It's worth more than my salary for a year."

On summer mornings, Ellard left home in a crisp seersucker suit, white shirt, and tie. In the evening, he arrived home wilted and dirty, often feeling so contaminated that he changed his clothes and shoes in the garage before coming into the house. Despite the bad working conditions, he was happy in his work.

And I was happy about our living circumstances and the friends we were making. There was plenty of good housing close to the medical center, and our first apartment looked too splendid to be true. When I first saw it I asked, "Who do we have to share the kitchen with?" To which Ellard replied, "Nobody, it's all ours." So now, with Ellard's salary of $4,200 a year, plus a small income of about a thousand dollars from his private patients, we began to buy furniture piece by piece, supplementing with furniture we made. We felt very settled and a part of the Baylor community.

The Baylor faculty members and their wives were warm and

welcoming. They lent us furniture while we were acquiring our own, took us on picnics at the beach on Galveston Island and entertained us at summer suppers in their back yards. The Baylor community functioned like a big family. The wives of the departmental chairmen were warmly supportive of the junior faculty wives and made sure that I was incorporated into the family.

I am still amused and amazed at my first encounter with Dr. DeBakey, the famous cardiovascular surgeon. We were invited to the DeBakeys' lovely home for dinner. When we arrived, Dr. DeBakey was standing near the entrance greeting the guests. I was expecting somebody tall and glamorous. Instead he was a small, rather homely man with a large, saber nose that revealed his Lebanese background. But he didn't seem small or unattractive very long. Walking over to me, he turned on all his charm, "My dear, I've been waiting to meet you!" Immediately he became ten feet tall and completely captivated me, a little assistant professor's wife. It was my first experience with Dr. DeBakey's charisma, a charisma that I was to observe and benefit from on many occasions – both professionally and personally. He was probably the major force that made Baylor a great medical school and he also became a good friend and support to our family.

The most surprising aspect of our move to Houston was Ellard's attitude about my working. There had been no discussion of it before we left Minnesota. After we got settled, Ellard broached the subject. I was expecting him to voice (again) his resentment about my letting work interfere with our marriage, but I was shocked. I must have succeeded in managing my work so well in Minnesota that he could not "tell that I was working," because now he said, "Why don't you go over to see the Chairman of Pediatrics to find out whether you could do some part-time work? You could get somebody to take care of young Ellard."

So, in September, two months after we moved to Houston, I went to see Dr. Russell Blattner, Chairman of the Department of Pediatrics, who told me that at the moment there was no opening in Pediatrics, but if he was awarded a grant renewal, he would have a part-time poliomyelitis research fellowship in January. He suggested that in the meantime there might be something I could do in the Department of Microbiology. Sure enough, Microbiology needed a teaching assistant, so each afternoon from 1:00 to 5:00 P.M., I assisted students in the laboratory. I also graded tests, and on one occasion, I was actually permitted to give a lecture. This experience in Microbiology was valuable; it was not only educational, but it also permitted me to meet faculty members with whom I would interact for years.

When January came, Dr. Blattner's research grant was renewed and he offered me a fellowship investigating the role of flies in the transmission of poliomyelitis. I was glad to work in polio research because it offered a possible opportunity to contribute to the control of this dread disease. Dr. Blattner's study was part of a nationwide effort to find ways to prevent polio. At this time, a number of investigators were working feverishly to develop an effective and safe vaccine, and in the meantime, efforts were being directed at other possible preventive measures.

It is difficult for anyone not growing up in the early 1950s to appreciate the enormity of the polio problem before the licensing of the Salk vaccine in 1955. When I was a child in the 1920s, polio was referred to as infantile paralysis because it affected mainly young children. By mid century, it was a disease not only of children, but also of young adults. In fact, the disease was more severe and had a higher mortality rate in adults than in children. Of all the diseases that I was to observe during my fifty years of medical practice, paralytic polio was the one that created the most terror. It struck the rich and poor alike, without warning, leaving patients paralyzed for life or dead within a few days.

Polio occurred sporadically year round, but the majority of cases occurred during large epidemics in the summer months. In 1951, there were over 10,000 cases of paralytic polio in the United States and in 1952, more than 21,000. Texas was so hard hit in 1950, that a special hospital annex, with iron lungs and other life-support equipment, had to be built at Jefferson Davis Hospital.

The reason for the seasonal incidence was not known. Did the virus become dormant in the winter? Was it harbored by insects? Was it transmitted by insects? If a reservoir (such as an insect) could be found, then a preventive approach could be designed. So from 1950 to 1952, I worked as a research fellow with

Dr. Charles Boyd who was already involved in Dr. Blattner's project.

Charles Boyd was a remarkable young man with indomitable spirit and optimism. A few years before I worked with him, while he was an intern, he had paralytic polio, stayed in an iron lung for about a year, and was left with complete paralysis of both legs and partial paralysis of his left arm. Despite this severe physical handicap, he was supporting his wife and children. Charles was wheelchair-bound, but with the use of his right arm and a little use of his left arm, supported in a sling, he designed protocols, kept meticulous research notes, and supervised a laboratory assistant. With the help of the assistant, he collected flies from the city dump, identified the various species, and learned to keep them alive under laboratory conditions. Before I joined the team, he and the assistant had also developed a functioning monkey colony. In 1950, tissue culture was not widely used for propagation of poliovirus, and in the Baylor laboratory all experiments had to be performed in monkeys.

My job was to isolate poliovirus from stool specimens of paralyzed patients. We needed the virus to feed to flies to see whether it multiplied within the flies or was merely transmitted on the body of the flies. After a number of steps in dealing with the patient specimens, I ended up with a clear, bacteria-free liquid that I hoped contained virus. Poliovirus, like most viruses, was not visible with an ordinary microscope, and it was impractical to try to detect its presence using an electron microscope, even if we had possessed one at Baylor (few institutions had electron microscopes in 1950). Working with liquid specimens was like trying to see the "emperor's clothing"; we were not sure we had anything until we tested it in monkeys. We inoculated a small portion of the liquid into a monkey and froze the rest. We inoculated the specimen through the nose (often provoking the monkey to sneeze) and also directly into the brain. While we carried out this dangerous work, we wore special clothing and plastic shields resembling welder's masks to protect us from the sneezes and from accidental splashes or spills.

Charles, who was very ingenious, adapted a dental drill for the intracranial injection. The lab assistant removed the monkey from the cage, wearing heavy gloves. We particularly feared bites because monkeys could carry a simian herpes virus that was fatal to humans. After the monkey was subdued, we anesthetized it, drilled a hole in the skull and then injected the specimen through a long needle into the brain. I always felt inhibited during this process because the other caged monkeys surrounding us seemed to understand the procedure and became highly agitated, gesticulating and screeching. Now came several weeks of daily monitoring of the monkey for signs of polio (loss of appetite, listlessness, fever, paralysis). We took the monkey's temperature daily – believe me, no small feat. If the monkey became ill, it was killed and a careful autopsy was performed to determine whether the classical lesions of polio were present and to culture specimens for poliovirus. Sometimes we could prove the presence of poliovirus. At other times, the monkeys proved to have tuberculosis, measles, or some other disease to which monkeys are susceptible.

When we finally proved the presence of virus, we were ready to infect flies with the positive specimens and then repeat all the arduous steps of injecting monkeys to determine whether the virus was present on the outside of the flies, whether it was in their bodies, and whether it had increased in amount within their bodies. Unfortunately, using a dissecting microscope, we found that flies were heavily parasitized by mites. Dr. Blattner was very excited about our findings, because early in his career he had proven that mites were the reservoir for St. Louis encephalitis virus. He imbued us with his enthusiasm and soon we were grinding tiny amounts of material composed of hundreds of mites, purifying another set of emperor's clothing, and injecting this into monkeys. Several times we, too, became excited, because some of the mite-injected monkeys became ill and died, but the cause of death always proved to be the result of something other than polio.

This slow, time-consuming, dangerous research took us two years (just a few years later, using tissue culture techniques, it would have required only a small fraction of that time). We learned that poliovirus could be transmitted on the bodies and in the excreta of flies, but we found that it did not multiply in either flies or mites, so we knew that neither flies nor mites were a reservoir for the virus. Our work, and that of others, indicated that humans were the only reservoir for poliovirus, and the seasonal incidence of polio epidemics remained unexplained as it still does today in the 1990s. The search for this answer was greatly reduced when a vaccine became available in 1955.

With the introduction of the Salk vaccine, given by injection, the number of cases of paralytic polio plummeted from approximately 20,000 to less than 1,000 per year, and with the use of the Sabin vaccine, given orally, the incidence dropped even more. By the decade 1984-1994, polio was virtually eradicated in the United States, with fewer than 10 cases per year (Melnick 1988).

I never thought that I would use any of the experience I gained working with poliovirus again, but the research later proved to be my introduction to virology and especially to the group of viruses to which poliovirus belongs, the enteroviruses. Today, the names of the enteroviruses are well known, polio, Coxsackie, and Echo, but in 1950, we were just beginning to learn about diseases due to this group of viruses. In later years, I was to spend a great deal of time working with diseases resulting from the enteroviruses, rubella virus and other viruses.

During the two years I did polio research, I had another small part-time job that kept me marginally in touch with pediatrics. I worked two half-days at Ripley House, a health center in one of the poorer areas of Houston. Here I performed physical examinations of children, gave immunizations, and got my first real introduction to urban poverty. Once a week I also attended Pediatric Grand Rounds at Jefferson Davis Hospital where I felt like a poor child with her nose pressed against the bakery window because I wanted to work with patients like the members of the faculty. I longed to be a real part of the Pediatric community.

Looking back, I wonder how I, who had been so goal-directed all my life, could get so far off the track in my career. I understand the compromises that I made during Ellard's sojourn in the army and in Minneapolis, but it is harder to understand why, if there was no Pediatric position for me at Baylor, I didn't go into practice in Houston. It was one of many times when I was doing the balancing act between career and family. This time, walking the tight rope between the two, I leaned more heavily toward family.

During our first few years in Houston, many things besides working were occupying my time. We were eager to enlarge our family, and in late 1950, our second son, John, was born. Just before he was born, we bought our first home, a $13,000 G.I. house that we could afford because the down payment was only $300, and the monthly payments were small. It was a three-bedroom, one-bath, cedar shakes house in a neighborhood of congenial young couples, and we loved it. It was located on a bald prairie then considered the edge of Houston (in reality 15 minutes from the medical center). And, of course, it didn't have expensive appliances, such as a dishwasher, garbage disposal, clothes washer and dryer, or air conditioning. Very few houses came with these conveniences; they were added as they could be paid for.

John was a calm, happy baby, a real joy, and he restored some of my confidence in myself as a mother. I worked in the polio lab until about a week before he arrived and was back at work a few weeks later. There was no such thing as any formal maternity leave, and I did not expect it. I was just lucky that Charles Boyd could continue our research while I was away from the lab. At home, we hired a part-time maid who was very good with the boys and life was going smoothly.

There was only one fly in the ointment – the prevalent attitude toward working mothers. Only a few women who did not have to work for financial reasons did so, and practically no faculty wives worked. Many women were openly hostile about my working. They made remarks such as, "You're a doctor's wife. Why are you working?" or "Doesn't your husband worry when you are out at night? (One of my clinics at Ripley House was held from 7:00 until 9:00 P.M.) My husband won't let me drive alone at night." Both my mother-in-law and my mother expressed extreme disapproval of my having a job outside the home. My mother-in-law's attitude was not surprising. She had been reared in a Quaker home that had strict role definitions. The man made the living and the woman ran home and catered to the man's every wish. But my mother's reaction was a shock; she did an 180-degree turn. The mother who had encouraged me so much in going to medical school now openly and constantly criticized my working and the way I dealt with my children. I dreaded letters and visits from both of our mothers.

Strangely enough, my father-in-law was enthusiastic and supportive of my working. He gave me a car so that I had transportation to work, and when he visited in Houston, I would find him reading want ads about housing and domestic help. He thought that we should have a house with servants' quarters and live-in help. He even offered to build us a larger house. I have often thought that he may have been right, but Ellard would never have considered it. He wanted a conventional wife in a home he himself could afford. He also demonstrated some embarrassment about having a working wife and began to refer to my work as "Martha's hobby." As a result, I began to diminish the importance of my work. At social affairs, I demurred when people commented that they understood that I was a doctor. My reply was something like, "Well, sort of." I felt compelled to add apologetically that I worked only part-time and had lots of time for my home and children.

Career women of today have trouble understanding this attitude, but the 1950s were very different from the 90s. Today, many women who stay at home as full-time homemakers apologize about not working outside the home.The fifties era was not an easy time to be a young mother and it was even harder to be a "working" mother. The mother's role was complicated by two factors: first, this was a time when young couples were establishing nuclear families. Having lived far from their homes during the war and having learned about other parts of the country, young people were leaving their extended families and losing the support of relatives. Second, it was a time of unrealistic idealism about the family. It was Ozzie and Harriet time, the baby boom era, the time when ads showed smiling mothers waxing kitchen floors wearing their pearls and high heels. In this atmosphere of the perfect, "togetherness" home, it was difficult for any mother to live up to society's expectations, and it was especially hard to be a "working" mother.

I felt beleaguered by all these influences – Ellard's feelings, the criticism of both our mothers, and society's attitude. I was exhausted from balancing my combined duties as super-wife, super-mom, and medical researcher, so when Dr. Blattner's polio grant expired, I decided to stop working for a while. I was pregnant again and I wanted to be rested and able to cope with a husband's busy career and three children under six, two of them less than two years old. Four months after I quit working, Cathy was born and she, too, was a calm, easy going, enjoyable baby. This time I stayed away from work for two years.

Memories of those two years are complex. On one hand, I enjoyed being with my children and helping my husband build his career. I was also having the opportunity to make many lifelong women friends. On the other hand, I resented the dichotomy in Ellard's life and mine. Each morning, Ellard went off to work resplendent in suit, white shirt, tie, and polished shoes. I, dressed for housework, got Ellard, Jr. off to kindergarten, and started washing clothes, hanging them on the line, washing dishes, cleaning house, and scrubbing the kitchen floor. During all of this I was watching my two toddlers. I was most resentful on garbage pickup days. Ellard and one of our doctor friends car-pooled. Ellard would pick up his colleague who lived down the street and come back by the house just as I was dragging out the garbage cans with two little children toddling behind me. The two men would wave cheerfully and I would mutter under my breath, "What am I doing taking out the G.D. garbage? My M.D. is just as damned big as theirs!"

My circumstances were no different from those of other young women in the neighborhood, but I adjusted less well than most of them. They seemed less frustrated than I felt. Perhaps it was because they were doing what they had always looked forward to doing, but I missed the mental stimulation of being with adults and sharing creative ideas. I can remember washing dishes and thinking, "I can't stand to think these same thoughts much longer. If I think them many more times I'll go off my rocker." And I missed reading, an impossible activity for a housewife with young children.

There are many surprises in rearing young children. Whoever thought that it would be hard to talk on the telephone or to take a bath? My friends and I used to laugh and dream of the day when we would once again be able to take a bath before our husbands came home. Since we were nuclear families, there were no relatives to help out when the mother was sick, to take the children to Sunday school, or just to take the children for a few hours to give the mother a brief respite. My neighborhood friends and I became a support group for each other and we drank lots of coffee surrounded by toddlers.

One thing that has not changed with time is the constancy required in taking care of toddlers. I have many memories of long rainy days with the children and me, shut in the house. I remember having a recurrent phantasy of a vast gymnasium where they could play and run off all their endless energy. I suspect that had day-care facilities existed, my children would have been frequent attendees. Many days of runny noses, diarrhea, and vomiting made me aware of the endless and repetitive duties of mothers with young children, and I like to think that my experiences made me a more understanding pediatrician in later years. Often my advice to worn-out, "nervous" mothers was to have adequate domestic help or to get a baby sitter, if at all possible. If this was my advice to them, why didn't I follow it myself? Simple. Our income didn't allow it. We were on a tight budget. Doctors in academic positions made small salaries forty years ago, and even today, those in nonsurgical specialties make considerably less than doctors in private practice.

One of the best things that happened to me was television. We got our first set in 1950 when there was only one TV channel in Houston, but soon there was the luxury of two more channels. I listened eagerly to the news reports. The children enjoyed cartoons, and Ellard and I relaxed looking at the night-time programs, good plays by wonderful authors such as Horton Foote, and comedy shows with Sid Caesar and Imogene Coca. I remember the McCarthy hearings in detail. They were a highlight in my life. Each day during the hearings I corralled the children in the living room with me, surrounded them with toys, and shut the door. The hearings were pure theater, and at night I had something adult and interesting to discuss with Ellard, something besides bottles and diapers and the vicissitudes of the day.

After two years of being at home full time, I realized that I was becoming seriously depressed. My self esteem was at a very low level. I had swallowed the myth of the perfect 1950s wife and mother, and both Ellard and I expected too much of me. The house had to be immaculate, the meals on time, the children well dressed, and I ran the house singlehandedly when Ellard was away on his numerous speaking trips. In addition, we frequently entertained visiting professors and their wives.

The good feelings that I had acquired in medical school about my worth as a woman and as a professional person had evaporated. Because I couldn't be perfect, I felt like a failure as a wife, as a mother, and as a doctor. In reality, I was a good wife and mother. I ran an orderly home, was a supportive wife, and a nurturing mother. It is sad that I could not feel successful in these roles. I lacked the confidence and self esteem to simply ignore others' opinions and to treat myself with more respect. I wish I could have done so. It would have been good for me, for Ellard, and for the children. In any event, I knew that I urgently needed to do something about my situation. I wanted to get back in to the mainstream of medicine, and with some trepidation, I told Ellard that I had to go back to work at least part time, and promised to do everything I could to save money so that we could pay for a maid. Somewhat reluctantly, he agreed knowing how unhappy I was.

Chpater 9

Return to Pediatrics

In 1954, I went to see Doctor Blattner again, this time not about a job, but about additional training in Pediatrics. I lacked four months of residency training to be eligible to take the American Board of Pediatrics examination. Certification by the Board was not essential for practicing Pediatrics, but it made one a bona fide pediatrician and that is what I wanted to be. I also needed to update my knowledge because I had been away from pediatrics for four years and the field had moved on rapidly.

Dr. Blattner and I worked out an arrangement whereby I would work as a resident half days for a year. He had no resident's salary for me so I agreed to work for nothing. Since I couldn't be available on nights and weekends, I wasn't able to work with hospitalized patients. My work was limited to daytime clinics, forcing me to learn about all aspects of pediatric medicine, not just serious problems. Not only was I getting updated in pediatrics, but I was becoming aware of the various community resources and learning how to use them.

I was very happy at work and things at home were going very smoothly, when tragedy struck. Ellard was diagnosed as having Hodgkin's disease, a malignant tumor of the lymph nodes. A year before, I had kept noticing an enlarged node on the left side of his neck. It wasn't painful, but at my insistence, he had it biopsied. When the biopsy specimen was examined, there was disagreement among several pathologists. Only one thought there was a malignant process; the others thought there was only a benign inflammatory reaction. Slides were sent to the Armed Forces Institute of Pathology, and there, too, a diagnosis of a benign process was made. So we relaxed about the matter.

However, in the fall of 1954, Ellard woke up one morning with a large swelling above his left collar bone. We were both horrified, because we knew that this was ominous. Ellard was admitted to the hospital, and a mass of lymph nodes was removed. This time there was no doubt about the diagnosis. The cells in the lymph nodes were typical of Hodgkin's disease – a cancer universally fatal at that time. (Today, the type of Hodgkin's disease Ellard had is curable.)

Ellard came home from the hospital feeling good physically, but with a very bad prognosis. We were told that his life expectancy was five years. We were stricken and drew close together, determined to give our unsuspecting young children normal childhoods as long as possible.

After a short course of x-ray therapy, Ellard went back to work as usual, except that he spent more time at home with the children and me. I, of course, continued to work, because it was clear that I was going to have to be in a good position to support the children and myself, and so Ellard and I were both more accepting of my being away from home. Now more gentle and supportive, Ellard told me that it was comforting to him to know that I would be able to earn a living.

Despite his prognosis, Ellard continued to be very busy. He was a marvelous physician, clinical researcher, and teacher. He worked long, hard hours at J.D. and consulted at other hospitals in Houston, all over Texas, and in hospitals in Louisiana and Oklahoma. Usually, he traveled by car, but on the longer trips, he was often transported in private planes sent by the patients' families. He was so respected for his sound judgment, that he was often asked to serve on committees, such as the building committee for the new Methodist Hospital that was to become a major teaching hospital for Baylor. And during all of this activity, he was writing and speaking at medical meetings all around the country.

At the end of my year of residency I needed a paying job and I had decided that I wanted to be a full-time academician in the Baylor Department of Pediatrics. This required expertise in some subspecialty area. The area that appealed to me was hematology. Dr. Robert Hettig, head of hematology in Internal Medicine at Baylor, offered me a fellowship (with pay!). However, when I asked Dr. Blattner whether, when I finished the fellowship, there would be an opportunity for me to join the department as the Pediatric hematologist, he told me that position would soon be filled by a young man who was studying with one of the Pediatric greats at Harvard. He added that he had one opening in the department – assistant to Dr. Bill Daeschner at J.D. There I would help run the general in-patient service but I would be expected to concentrate on infectious diseases. I was reluctant to be in the same subspecialty area as Ellard, who had been consulting on children as well as adults at J.D., but I was so thrilled to have a real place in the Department of Pediatrics that I seized it. Since I was not yet board eligible, I joined the department as an instructor, not in the usual beginning rank of assistant professor. I would work two-thirds time for a very meager salary, but at last, thirteen years after graduating from medical school, I was a real part of the pediatric community!

The night before I was to report to work I experienced a brief moment of panic. I realized that now the residents and students would be depending on me for the answers. I asked Ellard, "What will I do if they ask me something I don't know? Maybe they'll try to trip me up." He gave me strategic advice, "Just learn something about each pediatric problem and ask them about it before they ask you." I followed that advice and also learned to say, "I don't know, but that's a good question. Let's look it up," or "Please look that up and tell us about it tomorrow." Years later I heard an ex-resident say, "One thing I liked about Dr. Yow was that she could say, 'I don't know.'" I learned early on that you can't bluff residents!

When I reported to Bill Daeschner to find out my duties as his assistant, I thought that I would be under his wing, but I was quickly disabused of that idea. His injunction was, "You're on your own – don't follow me around!" He outlined my teaching schedule – bedside rounds, small seminars, and a few lectures.

Then he told me I would have the responsibility for children with infectious diseases in the isolation area on the tenth floor and on the sixth floor, the main pediatrics floor. Also I would provide consultations in the nursery on the fifth floor and in the pediatric outpatient department which was in a converted army barracks at one end of the parking lot.

While I was absorbing the rather large scope of my assignment, Bill advised me to develop some area of clinical research. His philosophy was that one could not be an outstanding teacher by merely teaching established dogma. In order to be a really fine teacher, one must be adding new knowledge. It was obvious from the very first day that Bill was glad to have me as an assistant and that he had absolutely no prejudice against women doctors. I could tell that we would be working together as equals.

After my indoctrination, Bill took me to see the small room that he and the residents were converting to a library on weekends, with Bill supplying the lumber and nails for the book shelves, of course. Next he took me around to the "office" of Dr. Murdina (Ina) Desmond. I knew Ina, but not very well. Her office was a 6 x 6 foot cubicle with a desk cluttered with papers and a microscope in the middle of glass microscope slides that seemed to have been tossed about helter-skelter by the wind. Here in the midst of this seeming chaos sat Ina at her microscope. She bounced out of her chair and gave me a hearty welcome. This was the beginning of a life-long friendship with Ina and a three-way camaraderie among Bill, Ina, and me.

Bill and Ina escorted me up to the 10th floor where my office was to be located. Bill was having a nurses' dressing room cleared out to serve as my office. It proved to be a long, narrow, dirty, odoriferous room with a scabrous window at the end. The window would have offered a beautiful view of Buffalo Bayou and downtown Houston, and some breeze into the unairconditioned building, but a sort of mottled grey and black plastic material was unalterably attached to it and the window was sealed shut. Undaunted, I saw the room as a wonderful combination office and laboratory. At J.D., there was no furniture available, so Bill advised me to go to the attic at Baylor, select some things, and requisition them. The best part of my new office/lab was its proximity to the large, bright, clean ten-bed isolation ward for children with infectious diseases. This ward had a million-dollar view of Houston. Never mind that it was in the middle of the psychiatry floor; it was mine and I could treat the patients. I hied myself over to Baylor, requisitioned an old desk, a worktable, and two creaky straight chairs. The Department of Microbiology lent me a small incubator and refrigerator, and I appropriated a pan and rack for staining slides and some bottles of stain. Ina lent me an old monocular microscope with the name M.E. DeBakey etched on the base.

My biggest problem was the lack of running water. The hospital might have piped some water in, but there was no way to put in a line for waste water. My solution to the problem was to install a five-gallon container of water with tubing and a stopcock on a shelf over the work table and to put a bucket for waste water under the table. At intervals, I went across to a psychiatry treatment room to wash my hands and to empty my staining tray. Finally I got into trouble – the psychiatrists wanted to know, "Who is that crazy woman who goes in and out of the shock room all of the time, and why is our sink purple?" I was evicted and forced to go further down the hall to a utility room, where bed pans were cleaned, to empty my waste bucket.

How can I describe those days in the 1950s at J.D.? There were down sides and up sides to working there. On the down side, J.D. was the typical metropolitan charity hospital – too small, underfinanced, underequipped, understaffed, impossible to keep clean because of overcrowding, and unairconditioned and stifling hot in the summer. Most of the patients were black, a few were Mexican-American and Caucasian; all were indigent. To qualify for care, patients had to be desperately poor, and this was before the advent of Medicare or Medicaid. I remember a period when to be eligible at J.D., a family had to have an income of less than $200 a month, regardless of the number of children. Even if the patients were seen in the clinic and had a drug prescribed, they might not be able to obtain the medicine because they had no money. The number of people needing care was overwhelming. An average number of 1,000 outpatients (adults and children) were seen per day, many sitting for long hours on hard benches waiting for their names to be called.

Over 100 pediatric patients came to the clinic daily, but only about 10 or fewer could be admitted to the hospital due to the shortage of beds. Many very ill children had to be managed as outpatients even though they should have been hospitalized. I was deeply concerned about some of the children we had to send home. These were children with parents who might be unreliable, parents who had no telephone to contact the hospital, or parents who had no transportation to bring the children back to the hospital if they got worse.

One early afternoon I got a call from a mother whose three-month-old baby sounded seriously ill. The mother said the baby's heart was racing, he was breathing fast and wouldn't take his bottle. I told her to bring him in and we would see him immediately. She replied that she had no transportation until night, that her husband was at work and she had no money. When I asked her to borrow some money from her neighbors and come on the bus, she said that she would try. I told her to tell them that we would give her money to repay them. About an hour later the woman, really only a girl, arrived with the baby who was ashen, limp, and in shock. We admitted him to the hospital immediately. He had paroxysmal auricular tachycardia, a problem common in adults, but relatively rare in infants and children. His heart rate was over 200 and he was in heart failure. The cardiologist came to see him immediately, prescribed a drug to slow the heart rate and told me that the infant could not have survived many more hours without treatment. I gave the young mother a little money to repay her debt to the neighbors, and the residents pitched in and gave her bus tokens so that in the future she could get to the hospital quickly. This was just one of many times when I saw the poorly paid house officers and nurses reach into their own pockets to help children and their families.

There is nothing new about people being unable to afford health care – nothing new about not having health insurance. The difference today from forty years ago is the public's awareness of the problem. Lack of affordable health care now affects middle income individuals so that they, and community and national leaders, now hear what fell on deaf ears in 1950s. Nor is there anything new about caring. Good health care workers have always been concerned and compassionate. The nurses and aides deserved medals for staying at J.D. when they could have made more money and had better working conditions in most other Houston hospitals. The dedication of the house officers was also outstanding. Intensive care facilities did not exist and special duty nurses were out of the question at J.D., so interns and residents spent long hours monitoring critically ill children.

On the up-side of working at J.D. was the tremendous opportunity to help people while gaining vast clinical experience. We saw not only large numbers of problems common to all children, but we also saw diseases that had become largely nonexistent in children who had received preventive care, such as whooping cough, diphtheria, tetanus, and tuberculosis. In this population, disease processes were frequently far advanced before the children were brought to the hospital with meningitis, lobar pneumonia, osteomyelitis, mastoiditis, severe diarrhea, terribly infected wounds.

Other than patients with infectious disease problems, there were children with rheumatic fever, nephrosis, rheumatoid arthritis, life-threatening malnutrition, battered children, children terribly wounded in accidents, rat-bitten children (faces almost destroyed, digits chewed off), children with lead poisoning, and in cold weather, children horribly burned by exploding heaters or fires stoked with kerosene. Frequently children were admitted to the hospital too late in the course of their illnesses to be saved. Not all of this was due to parental neglect or ignorance. Many parents had no immediate transportation or could not afford to miss work, so had to bring the children to the hospital after working hours.

Working at J.D. was often heart breaking, but a year's experience there was comparable to many years' experience in a smaller hospital with a more privileged clientele. I don't think a week ever passed that I didn't see some disease, or some variation of a disease that I had never seen before.

The "esprit´ de corps´" of the faculty and house officers was tremendous. Bill Daeschner, Ina Desmond, Aaron Mintz (director of the outpatient clinic), and I were the only Baylor pediatric faculty members based at J.D. Other members of the department were based at Texas Children's Hospital (TCH) and came to J.D. for weekly rounds and as consultants in crisply pressed clothes and polished shoes. But we four were the J.D.

crew, all young, energetic, wrinkled and hot. We worked side by side with the housestaff and students, trying to improve care for individual patients and trying to overcome the apathy of the community about health care for the poor. All four of us grew up during the depression in families short on money but long on resourcefulness and idealism. We were the perfect faculty for J.D., because it required coping ability.

Probably one of the things that the house officers appreciated most about the J.D. faculty was that we understood hard times, were genuinely concerned about their working situations and fought battles with the hospital administration to improve their lot. They appreciated Bill's providing space, lumber, and labor to make a library for them, and I suspect they considered my greatest contribution, maybe greater than teaching them infectious diseases, to have been getting the administrator to install a window air conditioning unit in their quarters located in the steaming hot hospital attic. I was empathetic – I knew what it was like to spend a southern summer in a hospital attic!

The faculty on the other hand appreciated the enthusiasm and dedication of the residents even when they were bone tired. During their training in the Baylor residency program, they rotated through both TCH and J.D., preferring J.D. where they were the patients' primary doctors instead of covering other physician's private patients, as they did at TCH. Those of us on the J.D. faculty supervised them, of course, but they had much more responsibility and autonomy at J.D. than at TCH.

I loved working with the residents at J.D. We struggled together, shared gratification over arriving at a difficult diagnosis or saving a desperately ill child, and we told funny stories and laughed at lunch time over soul food – turnip greens, pork chops, cornbread, and deep dish fruit pies.

I can count on the fingers of one hand the few residents who were motivated by wanting to make a lot of money (a motivation frequently ascribed to doctors by the public). Pediatricians are, in general, nurturing people, and they are concerned about the welfare of children. Those residents who worked with the poor learned early on that social situations are major determinants of the health of our nation's children. They learned that when a family is barely eking out an existence, a roof over their heads, food on the table, and clothes on their backs are the major concerns. Preventive health care is way down the list.

The thing I enjoyed most was seeing a new patient with the residents and students, collecting the necessary specimens from the patient, and then going into my little lab where we could look under the microscope and make a rapid diagnosis. We could have the answer more quickly, and frequently more accurately, than if we waited for the results from the hospital lab where we sent duplicate specimens. If a child was admitted with signs of meningitis – we could do a spinal tap, examine the fluid under the microscope, see the causative organism and start appropriate therapy in less than an hour. It was ideal for the patient and a wonderful learning experience for the residents and students.

The setup in the outpatient clinic was such that I could do the same kind of teaching there. One afternoon I was reviewing the case of a six-year-old with a rather glib medical student when he said, in a bored fashion, "Oh, this little girl just has impetigo," (a superficial skin infection due to streptococci or staphylococci). She did indeed have crusted lesions on her legs that looked like garden variety impetigo, but there were also a few unusual looking purple lesions around her ankles. Ordinarily I might have dismissed these as just a variation of impetigo, but since this was the only patient assigned to the student for the afternoon and because he had taken a sloppy, superficial history, I decided to make him work and learn something. I asked him what organism he thought was causing the sores. He replied, "Oh, streptococcus." On the basis of odds, he was probably right, but his casual attitude and his haste to escape clinic irritated me; so instead of just approving his note on the chart and prescribing the usual treatment for impetigo, I said, "I want you to take a specimen from one of these purple lesions, put it on a slide, stain the slide, and we'll look at it under the microscope to see whether there are strep alone or whether there are also staphylococci." Well, I learned as much or more than the student. I expected to see dark, blue, round organisms in grape-like clusters (staph) or dark, blue, round organisms in chains (strep). To my amazement, we saw pink, biscuit-shaped organisms in pairs, characteristic of the gonococcus (the bacteria that causes gonorrhea). This put an entirely different face on the matter. Now we knew that this little girl had been molested and that the gonococcus had entered through the genital tract, invading her blood stream and causing the lesions on her legs. A more thorough examination revealed a vaginal discharge loaded with gonococci. In this unusual case, we treated the child differently because of seeing the organisms under the microscope – both in the amount of penicillin we gave her and in an investigation of abuse.

Would I recommend culturing the skin lesions of all children with impetigo? No, but in dealing with the children who came to the clinic, I joined Aaron Mintz in urging the students to be as thorough as possible. They had more time than the busy residents trying to see large numbers of children. I explained to the students that it was important for them to do as much as they could for these patients, that the children might never have been to a doctor before and they might never come back again. Also, I stressed that the students should find out whether the children had been immunized. If not, at least we should start their immunizations. If they never came back, one dose of vaccines was better than nothing. When the students realized that not only were they there to learn, but also to be a part of the team trying to deliver health care under difficult circumstances, they responded with the idealism characteristic of most medical students and did a fine job. That's what working at J.D. was like – a constant learning process and a constant challenge to adapt to the special circumstances of the poor.

* * * * * * * *

A major aspect of my work that made life pleasant was my friendship with Ina. We worked together on sick newborns almost daily and we had an especially deep bond being among the few women M.D.s on the Baylor faculty. We also shared the problem of being working mothers and empathized with each other when we had to leave our own sick children at home to be taken care of by a maid. Our worst feelings came when our children woke up sick in the morning and we faced this conflict.

We didn't run into much prejudice against women at the hospital, but we dealt with a fair amount of patronizing behavior from some of the male members of the Pediatrics Department who spent most of their time at TCH. Bill Daeschner, Aaron Mintz, Ina and I all experienced some condescension from the TCH group. We were the J.D. crew and were considered to be from the other side of the tracks. Certainly, we made less money than the faculty based at TCH and because we were women, Ina and I got an extra share of the patronizing attitude, often actual bullying at the monthly departmental meetings. We hated those meetings but we developed a protective strategy. We were always well-dressed on those days and always had our hair and nails done; we had a touch of class and we sat next to each other so that we could nudge each other under the table as a reminder to resist saying anything controversial. We avoided any remark that would give the macho members of the group the opportunity to give us a response, such as "Well, you ladies get so upset over everything!" Too, we learned to handle everything possible with Dr. Blattner before the meeting by either an interview or letter so that our business would not be discussed during these vitriolic sessions.

One day, however, something came up to which I had to respond. When I did so the most macho man in the department said to me sarcastically, "Why don't you write one of your famous letters?" That became one of my and Ina's favorite quotes. When one of us complained too much to each other, the listener would say, "Why don't you write one of your famous letters?" We became expert at protecting our flanks, but often after these departmental meetings we were so frustrated that we went to lunch to defuse. On especially bad days we went shopping. We both loved beautiful clothes; Ina was big on hats and I on beautiful shoes. Somehow Dr. Blattner learned about our playing hooky and one day had me paged at Neiman Marcus about some trivial matter.

* * * * * * * *

Back on the home front, I was handling things better partly because I was happier and partly because we had moved to a larger home with adequate space in which the maid could work without being intrusive. The children were growing up and were less work and more fun. Ellard's health was robust, and for long periods of time, we actually forgot his diagnosis of Hodgkin's disease. In fact, our defense system was so good that, I think, we didn't really believe it. I was now able to balance work, carpools, and being a Cub Scout mother. My work schedule permitted me to spend valuable, good times with young Ellard, John, and Cathy. The only thing I had trouble fitting in was studying for my boards. I had completed the training requirements for the American Board of Pediatrics and after two years of practice at J.D., I would be eligible to take the exams.

When I discussed applying to take them, Ellard asked, "Why do you need your boards?" Obviously, he still had some resistance to the idea of my work being important to me or to the family. My answer was that I had decided to stay in academic medicine and that I would never be promoted without them. Eventually, I received the notice that I was scheduled to take the written exam in Houston and the oral exam in New Orleans in January 1957. Ellard was tough. His comment was, "Don't pay the $100 fee unless you intend to pass and remember the people who pass are those who study. I think you should plan to study at least four hours a day for six months."

So in July 1956, I began my studying. Sometimes this cut into my time with the children, but mostly, it cut into my sleeping time. My routine was to cook breakfast, get the children off to school, work at the hospital until three in the afternoon, spend time with the children, cook supper, supervise baths and homework, have children in bed by 9 o'clock, and then spend an hour with Ellard if he wasn't at the hospital or writing or traveling. I slept until 2:00 A.M., got up when the house was quiet and studied four hours. I jumped back in bed for a quick cat nap until it was time to get up and start a new day. Ellard kept tabs on me. He would ask, "Did you study four hours, yesterday? No? Well it's eight hours, today." You would have thought I was a school dropout. Ellard meant for me to pass! Weekends I didn't study. I just caught up on domestic things – mending, cooking, grocery shopping, errands. And usually we went out on Saturday nights. This was a frenetic pace, but there was a good feeling at night when we were all together, the children bathed and happy, having their allotted hour of television before bedtime. I remember the wonderful sense of thankfulness when they were tucked in bed and we were all together, safe and secure.

* * * * * * * *

Midway in my preparation for the boards, I realized that there were large gaps in my knowledge, gaps that could be filled only by some "round the clock" working in a hospital service and some uninterrupted study time. I knew that I couldn't manage this in Houston because my children would have inadequate care. It occurred to me that the Carolina relatives might be willing to keep the children two months during the summer and let me go to Duke University Hospital for some intensive training. This way I could live at the hospital, but be nearby should the grandparents need me. Ellard and I discussed this and he reluctantly agreed to my pursuing the matter. The North Carolina grandmother Yow agreed to take John, and my sister and mother in South Carolina said they would be glad to have young Ellard and Catherine. Now I had to find the money for my expenses.

Dr. Blattner had the Jesse Jones Fellowship Fund that permitted him to send residents to other training programs for brief periods. Generally the residents went to Boston Children's Hospital, but Dr. Blattner was willing to give me the usual $500 to go to Duke. This covered the transportation of the children and me to the Carolinas and Duke provided my room and board.

As the time to leave home and to be separated from Ellard neared, I became more and more anxious. I had tremendous conflict that was aggravated by Ellard's thinly disguised disapproval of the undertaking and by knowing that I would miss him and the children terribly. I paced the floor at night. One day I was going. The next I was staying at home. Finally D-Day arrived and I went.

When Dr. Jerome Harris, Chairman of the Department of Pediatrics at Duke, asked me how I envisioned spending my time at Duke, I told him that I didn't want to be an observer, that I wanted to actively work on the service. I added that I felt it would be difficult for me to be a resident because I didn't know how to get anything done in a new place, and that I would do better as an intern under the guidance from the residents. So now, although I had already been on the faculty at Baylor for two years, I was back at the bottom again. I must have been crazy. This was, indeed, the best way for me to learn but it almost killed me. When I had been an intern at Bowman Gray twelve years before, I was twenty-two and the youngest intern in the hospital. Now I was thirty-four, the oldest intern at Duke, and my stamina was considerably reduced. I hadn't realized the difference in resiliency that twelve years could make. Every time I sat down I had to fight falling asleep.

The Duke house officers were my salvation. They welcomed me into the trenches, dubbed me "The Yellow Rose of Texas" and included me in their social activities. Duke, like Baylor, was one big family.

That is not to say that Dr Harris was not a hard taskmaster. He was a bachelor and was ever-present in the hospital. He made sure that we worked hard, frequently showing up on the wards at midnight. When he wasn't on the wards, he was in the library, acutely aware of whether we were there studying as he expected us to do on our nights off. He had the habit of many attending physicians, including me at J.D., of saying to the interns and residents, "It would be interesting if you would do some extra investigation into this case." I, bone tired, thought bitterly, "If it's so interesting why don't you do it yourself?" When I returned to my job at Baylor, I never said it to a house officer again.

I never let Dr. Harris know that I had any expertise in infectious diseases because I wanted to concentrate on other aspects of pediatrics that summer. The last week I was at Duke, I identified something under the microscope that had the house officers stumped and Dr. Harris asked, "How do you know that? If you are an expert in infectious diseases, why haven't you let us know?" I felt like, saying "No way, Jose, you would have worked me to death!"

* * * * * * * *

Yes, I did pass my boards. Back in Houston, I took the written part of the examination, which was very hard but not frightening. Having passed that hurdle, I was off to New Orleans for the oral exams. I was terrified. Each candidate would have four examiners and must be approved by three of the four. Bill Daeschner tried to reassure me by telling me that it was just a chance to be with the greats. I didn't feel that way. One of my fears was that I would get examiners who didn't think women should be in medicine. The toughest examiner was said to be Dr. Ralph Plateau from Tulane and if you got him, you were dead!

On the morning of the exam I spent a long time in my hotel room trying to decide how to dress so I would look professional, but not masculine. I donned a beautiful brown suit, pearls, small gold earrings, an antique gold bracelet, and topped it all off with a small mink cape, an encouragement gift from my supportive father-in-law. As I walked the two blocks to Tulane, I began to worry that the examiners would think me frivolous. One by one, the adornments came off – earrings, pearls, bracelet, and when I got to the waiting room, the mink cape. The mink came off because I was afraid the academician examiners would think I made too much money. Big joke!

When I was summoned to the inner sanctum, I left the mink on a chair in the waiting room, fully aware that it might be stolen but thinking, "To hell with the mink!" The first of my examiners welcomed me into his office with, "Come in. I'm Ralph Plateau." Somehow, I got through the interview, but I made some really big mistakes and I emerged thinking, "That's it. I'm dead!" I muddled through the sessions with the next two examiners, but the fourth threw me a curve. He used the first part of the period quizzing me and then he said, "That's enough. Let's talk about some more general things. How do you feel about being a woman doctor? Would you advise your daughter to go into medicine? What do you think about women doctors getting married?" Now I was panicked. What did he want to hear? How did he feel about all these things? My overriding thought was that I had to be tactful and as low key as possible. I replied that I liked being a doctor and found it very gratifying. I was less positive about the next question. Yes, if my daughter truly wanted to be a doctor, I'd encourage her, but I would tell her it was a very hard road. And what about marrying? Yes again, but she would need to choose her husband very carefully. My questioner seemed satisfied, and relieved my anxiety by telling me that his daughter was a doctor and had just gotten married.

Next, I was sent back to the waiting room with the other nervous fellow candidates until the examiners decided whether to question us further. Being called back in meant you were on the borderline. If you were not called back you had either passed or had totally failed. After a short time, a secretary came out and dismissed me. I left not knowing whether I had passed or failed. I picked up the mink, and with one of my fellow sufferers, went to the nearest cocktail lounge. Two weeks later I received a congratulatory letter and for the first time felt like a bona fide pediatrician. Ellard was proud of me and I knew I had his blessing when he said, "Now that you have your boards, I think you should have a mending woman. You can't do everything." Not only that, he hired a back door garbage pick up service!

Six months later, I was promoted to assistant professor at the same time Ellard became a full professor. In the seven years we had been in Houston, Ellard had a meteoric rise from assistant professor to associate professor to full professor. During that same time, I had a long uphill pull from fellow to assistant professor. Did I resent this difference? No, I can honestly say that I really didn't think about it. I was proud of him and I knew that by relieving him of domestic responsibilities and by being a good faculty wife and hostess, I had played a major role in his success. With his prognosis of a short life, I wanted his life to be as happy and full as possible.

Chapter 10

An Epidemic Becomes A Catalyst for Change

SUDDENLY, WHEN I HAD BEEN an assistant professor only a few months, my quiet job at J.D. changed dramatically. Though I was busy, my job was low key. I was teaching, seeing patients, beginning research in bacterial meningitis. I still had no secretary, no real laboratory, no laboratory technician, and was so low on the totem pole that I was not serving on any committees. Then, as would be true of the rest of my career, the emergence of a major infectious disease problem decided the course of my work and really changed my life.

In the latter part of the 1950s, a great epidemic of antibiotic-resistant staphylococcal infections occurred throughout the world, and our hospital was especially involved. Now it was essential for me to work full-time at the hospital, and since I was working on the problem side-by-side with Ellard, he understood my being away from home from eight to five and sometimes at night. Although the children were young, they understood about the epidemic, and I heard them discussing it with their friends. They were obviously proud of having a father and a mother who were contributing to the community. This was a turning point in my career. I was no longer apologetic about being a working mother. Now I felt free to work to my full ability and thoroughly enjoy it.

What was the staphylococcal epidemic and why did it occur? The bacterium, *Staphylococcus aureus*, commonly called staphylococcus or just staph, was not a new organism. It has plagued man for hundreds of years and still does today. There are many strains of the organism and these strains are ubiquitous. Their natural habitat is the human nose where they are normal flora and usually cause no harm. They are hardy bacteria and can exist for long periods in dust, bed clothes, carpets, and on other objects. Some strains establish themselves in the nose more readily than others, and some are more pathogenic (have greater ability to cause disease). The most common problems due to the staphylococcus are skin infections, such as boils, carbuncles, or abscesses, but the organism can invade the blood stream and can cause infection in any organ of the body. Wherever it occurs, it causes destruction of tissue and the formation of pus. This pus is teeming with bacteria that, if not properly handled, can contaminate the environment.

If this was a common organism well known to the medical profession, what caused a sudden and massive epidemic? Multiple circumstances produced the epidemic; changes in the staphylococcal organisms present in hospitals, changes in hospitalized patients, and changes in hygienic practices within hospitals.

When penicillin became available in the mid-40s, virtually all of the strains of staphylococcus were susceptible to penicillin. We used penicillin and newer antibiotics to manage almost all infections, so that large amounts of antibiotics were used, often indiscriminately. By the mid-50s, about 30% of the strains of staphylococci within hospitals in the United States (and in other developed nations) were resistant to penicillin and other antibiotics.

It seems strange that the medical profession was not more vigilant about these changes, but after a decade of using antibiotics, doctors were just becoming aware of the intricacies of bacterial ecology. Infectious disease experts had warned that penicillin-resistant staphylococci existed in nature and could emerge as prevalent strains, but little attention was paid to these predictions. Now as we removed the antibiotic-sensitive strains, resistant strains were increasing and replacing the sensitive ones. It was similar to destroying the balance of nature in the animal world; destroy the cats and the rats increase or kill the birds and the insects increase.

Not only were the organisms in the hospital changing, but so were the patients. Because of medical advances, the number of patients who were particularly susceptible to infection was increasing. Younger and younger premature infants were surviving. The number of the elderly was increasing as people were living longer with debilitating diseases. Cancer chemotherapy was altering the immunity of patients with malignancies. Surgeons were performing more complex procedures that interrupted the body's natural barriers, using indwelling intravenous lines and installing prosthetic devices, such as artificial heart valves and aortic patches, devices that easily became infected.

The dependence on antibiotics to cure all infections lulled the medical profession into a false sense of security, and infection control procedures within hospitals were relaxed. There were fewer facilities for isolation of infected patients, personnel were less careful about gowning, masking, and hand washing. Housekeeping practices, such as careful cleaning of rooms between patients, became lax.

Now onto this stage ripe for problems, "hot strains" of staphylococci (strains identified by complicated typing as "phage type 80/81") entered the hospitals. These type 80/81 strains had all the characteristics to make them dangerous; they had the ability to spread easily from patient to patient; they were efficient colonizers entering the noses of hospital personnel and patients making them carriers; and they were virulent, causing severe tissue destruction and frequently invading the blood stream. Many patients who escaped staphylococcal disease in the hospital carried the bacterium home and developed infections several weeks later. They also spread it to their family members and throughout the community.

J.D. was particularly hard hit. The first evidence of the problem in our hospital occurred in 1956 in the large, crowded, understaffed newborn nursery with a small outbreak of staphylococcal infection. Ellard helped Ina bring this under control using a new antibiotic, novobiocin, with which he was working in his lab. There was a brief reprieve, but in 1957, another 80/81 staphylococcal outbreak struck J.D. in full force. This organism was resistant to novobiocin, as well as to penicillin, tetracycline, and streptomycin. Infections were rampant in the nursery. Also, patients on other services were becoming infected, but in smaller numbers, and in most cases with less dire effects. Ellard was aware of the problem on the internal medicine wards, but most of the physicians on other services, such as surgery and obstetrics practiced tremendous denial. They did not want to admit their patients were infected.

It was impossible to adopt such an attitude in the nursery. Infants were covered with staphylococcal pustules, many had breast abscesses, and others had massive infection of the umbilical area destroying the abdominal wall. In many cases, the organism entered the blood stream causing pneumonia, bone infection, and meningitis. These babies were riddled with infection and many died.

Ina was having a terrible time. She was responsible for the enormous nursery service, about 9,000 infants per year (24 newborns per day). Many of these infants were sick, and the rate of prematurity was high, because only 50% of their mothers had received prenatal care and had been sick or undernourished themselves. The nursery was too small for this influx of babies each day, and the bassinets had to be crowded together (much closer than recommended for infection control by the American Hospital Association). Sinks were not convenient for hand washing. There was inadequate space for isolation of sick infants and there were too few nurses, attendants, and housekeeping personnel. There were not even enough linens or diapers. Ina worked long and hard to get these problems remedied, but with little success.

I was working with Ina treating the babies who developed staphylococcal disease while they were still in the nursery, but I was even busier with one- to two-week-old infants who had been in the nursery briefly, had been colonized by the epidemic organism, and developed illness after they went home. Now they reappeared in the clinic or emergency room and had to be admitted to a special isolation area on the pediatric floor under my care.

These were terribly ill children, and the residents and I labored long and hard to save them. We had to use antibiotics difficult to administer to infants and children that had generally been abandoned for use at any age, because of their side effects. Whenever possible, we drained infected areas since this hastened recovery. We did many procedures ourselves when the surgeons couldn't come promptly. We drained deep abscesses, joints, and chest cavities. We even tapped the pericardial sac around the heart and instilled antibiotics. When I think back, I can hardly believe the things we did, things we (as pediatricians) probably wouldn't do today for fear of litigation. Today we would wait for a surgeon, but then we saved many children who otherwise would have died. Working with these terribly ill children, the residents and I formed a strong bond and when I see them at medical meetings forty years later, we greet each other with warm affection and reminisce about our struggles during the staph epidemic.

Ina and I worked feverishly trying to enlist the aid of administrators at the hospital and at Baylor in controlling the problem. We met apathy, actual disbelief, and condescension. Our hand-delivered letters were not even answered. The attitude was that we were hysterical women. Ina was more immediately involved, so she bore the brunt of these responses. Somebody in the medical school administration even went so far as to con the chairman of the Department of Psychiatry into trumping up an excuse to drop by Ina's office to assess her mental stability. She was enraged! On another occasion at a meeting with the obstetricians, one of them on hearing her report of the breast abscesses, allowed in a thick twangy Texas drawl, "Aw, you haven't got an infections problem. There's just a pervert in the nursery fooling with the babies' breasts." Ina didn't tell me about the latter incident until many years later. By then, it was hilariously funny to me, and when I asked her why she hadn't told me at the time, she said she was too angry and humiliated to discuss it. The surgeons said we were tilting at windmills. I think there was little doubt that the reason we were ridiculed and could get nothing done about the situation was that we were women and pediatricians, neither of whom had much clout at the medical school.

Soon infants began dying in alarming numbers, and Bill Daeschner joined us in the campaign for additional nursery space and personnel to provide isolation. Now we gained credibility, but there was still no cooperation from the hospital or the medical school. Finally, in desperation, the three of us, Ina, Bill, and I, put our jobs on the line and took a daring step. We declared the nursery unsafe and notified the hospital administrator and the dean of the medical school that the nursery was closed to all further admissions. Infants were being born at a rate of about one per hour and there was nowhere for them to be housed. This, of course, forced a crisis in Obstetrics, and the obstetricians who had been indifferent to the problem were forced to face it. Within the hour we got action! It was like watching hot water being poured on an ant bed. Activity was intense. The dean of the medical school, the hospital administrator, and the chairman of obstetrics appeared at the nursery and summoned Ina, Bill, and me to accompany them on a tour of possible alternative facilities. They offered us several broken down, totally inadequate areas that we promptly rejected. One was a part of an old tuberculosis hospital in a group of old abandoned frame shacks with vines growing in through the cracks. At the end of a long day when they realized that we were adamant about providing a real solution to the problem, they mobilized a whole building that adjoined the hospital and was virtually unused. Obstetrical facilities and new nurseries were operational in no time at all. In order to prevent introduction of the epidemic strain of staphylococcus to the new unit, no infants in the old unit were transferred to the new facility, and no nurses harboring the organism in their noses were assigned to work there.

Since Ellard was the head of infectious diseases at Baylor, the dean appointed him to coordinate the efforts to control the epidemic. It was a wise move, because Ellard had wonderful organizational ability. The first thing he did was to establish a hospital infections control committee, one of the first in the nation. He realized that to solve such a massive problem, the cooperation of many services was essential. The committee was composed of representatives from all the medical and surgical services, the nursing service, housekeeping, engineering, and all other ancillary services. This was a stroke of genius. Without the help of all these groups, nothing could have been accomplished. The next step was to call for assistance from the city and state health departments and the National Centers for Disease Control (CDC) in Atlanta.

The response and cooperation were remarkable. Within forty-eight hours, personnel from the CDC were present. Their first recommendations were methods to assess the magnitude of the problem and to determine the possible sources of the staphylococcus and how it was being spread. These included observation of hospital procedures, review of housekeeping policies, study of the air flow within the hospital, measuring the number of organisms in the air in various areas – the nurseries, the operating rooms, the obstetrical suite, the wards, the halls, the elevator, and the linen room. This meant hundreds of cultures.

When the enormity of the task was realized, it was clear that the already overburdened hospital laboratory could not handle the massive amount of bacteriologic work that was required. Ellard's small research laboratory was pressed into service, but it was inadequate. So Mr. Ben Taub, chairman of the hospital board, gave Ellard money to remodel an old machine shop into a laboratory where new antistaphylococcal antibiotics could be studied. I was given a laboratory in the new Ob-Nursery building. The state provided money for a technician in my lab and the CDC supplied me with two epidemiology nurses and a secretarial salary. The director of the City Laboratory assumed the monumental job of preparing the organisms we isolated for typing by the CDC, and one of the professors from the Department of Microbiology at Baylor performed all the air sampling techniques.

This maelstrom of activity did not go unnoticed by the media. Since J.D. was a public facility, the epidemic became a political football. The newspapers published lurid headlines: "Babies Still Dying at Jefferson Davis Hospital," "Hospital Guilty of Cover Up." Gradually the reporters began to mention the fact that the size and budget of the hospital were woefully inadequate for a community the size of Houston and Harris County, and that crowding and inadequate numbers of personnel contributed to the problem. The two major Houston newspapers were so persistent in sensational reporting and so competitive in getting the day-by-day head count, that we had to issue a daily report from the administrative office. This had to be timed so that we were fair to both the morning and afternoon papers. The reporters became so troublesome so that I often walked up and down ten flights of stairs and slipped in and out of the back of the building to avoid them. This type of harassment continued for almost a year. Our home phone rang persistently day and night. It was so disruptive that at intervals we had to take the family out of town for the weekend to get some rest.

By the time the investigation of the epidemic was begun, it was not possible to identify any single source for the epidemic organism or any single factor in its spread. There were multiple sources. The organism was found in all parts of the hospital. Large numbers of patients and personnel were found to be carriers, equipment was contaminated, air sampling showed that the two areas with the highest bacterial counts were the operating room and the elevator. A study of the air circulation in the hospital revealed that the air from the autopsy room was exhausted across the clean linen room.

With the situation well-defined, a massive control program was instituted, but the epidemic raged on. Surgical patients developed wound infections; eighty-six postpartum women developed breast abscesses that lasted for months and sometimes destroyed as much as a third of the breast tissue; and hospital personnel became infected. The chief hospital engineer almost lost his scalp to multiple, undermining abscesses; numerous residents and staff members had boils and carbuncles and had to be removed from duty. It was almost a year before the epidemic could be brought under control. In the meantime, 324 individuals had staphylococcal disease, 123 of these were newborn infants, and 201 were older children and adults. Many of the 324 had prolonged illnesses and 27 died. This was a terrible staphylococcal outbreak, probably the worst of the entire nationwide epidemic.

There were, however, several positive effects of this disaster. It welded the hospital staff into a cohesive working group; it established a hospital infection control committee as essential to all hospitals; it led to the study of new antistaphylococcal antibiotics; and most important, it opened the eyes of the Houston community to the urgent need for a new, larger, and better equipped hospital, and it was the catalyst for change, albeit slowly.

On a personal level, it was a valuable experience for me. I feel guilty when I say that I benefitted from such a terrible catastrophe, but it did, indeed, change my career. Our roles in controlling the epidemic brought Ellard and me back to working together as we had in our house officer days. He invited me to join him in assessing a new antibiotic, kanamycin, in the treatment of staphylococcal disease. He studied the drug in adults, and I, in children. It was highly effective and responsible for saving many lives.

I remember the first infant that I treated with kanamycin – a three-month-old girl critically ill with staphylococcal pneumonia. I was not sure about the optimal dose to use, and I was frightened about possible side effects, but knew she would not survive very long without some effective therapy. The resident, Dr. John Jones, and I had tried every other available antibiotic, and all had failed. Kanamycin was all we had. We started the drug early one morning and John stayed by her side for the next twenty-four hours. I was awake all night, and by 5:00 A.M. was back at J.D. When I arrived at the bedside, John, tired and unshaven, was all smiles. The patient was responding. That little girl made history. Her chest x-rays appeared in numerous articles. For the next several years, kanamycin was the drug of choice for staphylococcal infections.

Kanamycin was the first antibiotic I ever studied in depth. It was effective against a number of bacteria other than staph, and I used it extensively and carefully assessed its side effects. In 1958, both Ellard and I were invited to present papers describing our experiences with kanamycin at The New York Academy of Sciences. Ellard had been presenting papers for a decade, but this was my first presentation, and my first trip to New York. I was understandably nervous and practiced my presentation many times. I planned to be very formal but when the moderator, an army colonel, introduced me by saying something about my being a southern belle and having a charming southern accent, I responded, "I had planned to start my talk by saying 'Ladies and Gentlemen' but instead I will just say, 'Cunnel and You-all.'" The ice was broken and my talk was a great success. It was a heady experience!

The New York trip was followed by a trip to San Francisco where Ellard and I gave papers before The American Medical Society, and our work was reported in *Newsweek*. I was so excited about these experiences that the residents teased me by calling me "The Kanamycin Kid."

Now I took another personal step forward. I went on a speaking trip without Ellard. I was invited to present our experiences in treating children with kanamycin at the International Pediatric Conference in Montreal. Ellard was not happy about my going (he had never kept the children before) and doing so was hard in the face of his disapproval, but go I did.

Dr. Blattner, Mrs. Blattner, Ina, and I went together and had a marvelous time. The sponsor for my trip was Bristol Myers, and my host was a handsome, suave Frenchman with impeccable manners. He entertained our group royally and was so protective of me that he would hardly let me carry my purse. He reminded me of Rozzano Brazzi in *South Pacific*, and when I was with him I heard the strains of "Some Enchanted Evening." He treated me like a princess, and I basked in the warmth of his attentions. The Blattners were highly amused, and Ina, my roommate, acted in her careful Scottish way. She was perturbed and kept close check on my activities. She was afraid I had gotten out-of-hand, but I had a splendid, innocent, carefree time. When I returned to Houston, I had a cool reception. But there was still enough of the glow of the trip left for me to be able to survive the coolness without being upset, until about a week after my return when Ellard confronted me with a bounced check. Oops! I was feeling so great when I checked out of the Queen Elizabeth Hotel in Montreal that I had signed the check, not Martha Yow, but Queen Yow. It took me a long time to live that one down!

The staphylococcal epidemic not only thrust me onto the national scene, but it also launched me locally. I was asked to consult at a number of Texas hospitals that were having nursery outbreaks of staphylococcal disease, and I think it was at this time I began to be viewed as an expert in infectious diseases and in antibiotic management. Certainly it was then that I began to work at Texas Children's Hospital as well as at J.D. and to consult at other Houston Hospitals. Ellard encouraged me to do so, saying, "It's not fair for you to use your expertise to help only the poor. You should work with private patients, too."

After the staphylococcal epidemic subsided, Ellard and I continued to work together, studying promising new antibiotics. He in adults, and I, in children. We also worked together when we joined other doctors at J.D. in mounting a community campaign to build a new hospital and to establish a taxing district to provide adequate funding. We spoke to church groups and civic organizations and published editorials in the Houston newspapers. This was an all out effort, and in the early sixties, the voters approved the taxing district and a new city-county hospital, the Ben Taub General Hospital, which was built in the medical center adjacent to Baylor.

After the staphylococcal epidemic subsided, I never went back to working alone. I was able to obtain funding to keep the core members of our staphylococcal team together. The funding came from small grants supported by pharmaceutical companies to study new antibiotics and a large grant from the National Institutes of Health (NIH) to study infantile diarrhea, a major cause of serious illness and death at our hospital.

The purpose of the NIH grant was to determine the causes of diarrhea, both bacterial and viral. Dr. Joseph Melnick, a world renowned virologist and Chairman of the Department of Virology and Epidemiology at Baylor, agreed to be co-investigator on the project (Melnick 1988). In fact, his name on the grant application undoubtedly played a large part in my receiving it. I was responsible for the patient care and bacteriologic studies and he for the virologic portion of the investigation. Working with Joe was a wonderful educational experience. From him I learned about study design and analysis of data, and I learned about decisiveness. He was probably the most decisive, efficient person I ever knew. One day, when I asked him how he made so many rapid decisions, he replied, "It's better to make 100 decisions and have 5 of them wrong than to make none at all." That statement became a motto for me.

Meanwhile, I was developing a pediatric infectious disease section. My dream was to have a section with faculty members expert in bacterial diseases, virus diseases, and immunologic problems, and a program with several fellows in training at all times. The fellows would be individuals who had completed their pediatric residency and wanted to become specialists in infectious diseases.

Once, as a child, I heard my mother talking in awed respect about someone who had received a fellowship. When I asked her what a fellowship was, she said, "It's sharing between a teacher and an advanced student where each helps the other and they are in fellowship with each other." I never forgot that explanation and it expressed my feelings about the interaction between my fellows and me.

In the early sixties, I was awarded an NIH fellowship grant, and our team (my secretary, technician, research nurse, two fellows, and I) moved to a great laboratory in a new research wing at Baylor and now we were off and running. I was still the only faculty member and I made rounds with one fellow at Ben Taub in the mornings and with the other at Texas Children's Hospital in the afternoons, but we were on the way to being a real Pediatric Infectious Disease Section, one of the first in the nation.

Chapter 11

The Hardest Balancing Act

IN 1960, LIFE WAS REALLY going well for us. We were enjoying our work and our home. Our children were well and happy and at wonderful ages – eight, ten and thirteen; the ages when all could get themselves into the car but no one could drive it. We had a full social life with Houston friends and interesting visitors from many places – mostly scientists and musicians. We were in the prime of life; I was thirty-seven and Ellard, forty-one. Then a terrible blow fell when, in September, Ellard and I were on a deep sea fishing weekend at Port Isabel on the Texas coast. About 1:00 A.M. on Sunday, Ellard awoke with agonizing abdominal pain. He diagnosed his problem as gall bladder colic, and we immediately left for home. He lay on the back seat in severe pain as I drove the three hundred miles to Houston.

Nothing ever looked so good as the entrance to The Methodist Hospital when we arrived. We were met by our good friend, Dr. Stanley Crawford, who immediately took Ellard to the operating room. As the stretcher was being wheeled by, Stanley stopped to tell me that he thought that Ellard's pain was, indeed, gall bladder colic, but he reminded me that we had to consider it might be something else. I was oblivious to any other possibility and went calmly to the waiting area for families of surgical patients. After a long while, Stanley came to tell me about the surgery. Ellard didn't have gall bladder disease. The colicky pain was the result of compression of the common bile duct of the gall bladder by enlarged lymph nodes. The Hodgkins disease had spread and there were enlarged lymph nodes throughout the abdomen. When Stanley told me, it was as though an enormous sledge hammer had struck the top of my head, and I fell to the floor in a dead faint.

The news of Ellard's illness traveled like wild fire through the medical center and friends rallied to our aid even before Ellard came out of the surgical recovery room. Dr. Bob Hettig, a close friend, had diagnosed Ellard's disease as Hodgkins seven years earlier and, of course, would continue to be his physician. Dr. Ed Ory, who worked with Ellard part time in infectious diseases and who also was one of our closest friends, would join Bob Hettig in treating Ellard when the inevitable life-threatening infections occurred. In the meantime, he would assume many of Ellard's academic duties. His wife, Norma, came to the hospital immediately to offer me help with the children or whatever I needed. All of our friends gathered round, and I felt that loving arms were supporting me and my family.

After the operation Ellard and I faced the terrible truth, grieved together and began to make plans. Now we had to tell our families and friends that he had Hodgkins. Our parents needed to know the bleak prognosis. We would tell our children, too, but we would not tell them how serious it was because they were still so young. We knew that Ellard would have a long period of convalescence from the extensive surgery and then a period of x-ray therapy, but we hoped he would be able to go back to work late in the fall. In the meantime, his associates would carry on his work. With his usual optimism, Ellard began to think of the best ways to spend happy and constructive time with the children and me.

He told me, "The first thing I want to do when I get up is to buy a small place on the water so that we can spend time with the children sailing, fishing, and just being out of doors. It needs to be close enough to Houston that we can use it year round, but we need to be away from the telephone and interruptions so we can have some close family life." Then we had to talk about his future travel plans for speaking engagements. He wanted to keep these to a minimum, but while he was in the hospital, he received an invitation for an expense-paid trip to Italy and Switzerland in September of 1961, a year away. He said that he didn't know what to reply. This time I was stalwart. "Write the organizing committee that you will do it. We're going!" We did both of these things; bought a beach house and went to Europe.

Ellard was discharged from the hospital about three weeks post surgery to continue his convalescence at home and to receive x-ray therapy as an outpatient. The x-ray therapy was a bad experience. He received it Mondays through Thursdays and then was given a reprieve over the weekends. On Mondays he felt good, but within forty-eight hours after the treatment was resumed, he became nauseated and terribly depressed. He just lay and stared at the ceiling. Then each weekend he returned to his natural affect. Those depressed days when he couldn't eat and lay almost inert were awful for him and for the family. He lost weight and was terribly weak. Eventually, the course of x-ray was over and he began to recover.

By November, he was able to lie on the back seat of the car for short trips and even before he was able to go to work, we began our search for a beach house. Our friends, Ed and Norma Ory, made this search possible by driving us to look at possibilities, Ellard lying on the back seat of the car with his head in my lap. Ed, Norma, and I did the initial survey of potential places and helped Ellard out of the car to look at a selected few. On a cold, misty Saturday afternoon in December, we found a sparsely populated area on West Galveston Island, Jamaica Beach, where the island was only two miles wide between the ocean and the bay. There were about fifteen houses built up on stilts and three on the ocean side were for sale. Ellard said, "You all look at them and choose the best one for me to look at. I can only go up the steps at one place." That's what we did. The chosen house was small, but it had a big combination living room, dining room, and kitchen that stretched across the front and offered a broad sweeping view of the ocean. It was such a contrast to the dark, closed up, old fashioned beach cottages that we had been shown that we were instantly taken with it. That night when we discussed the house I commented that I didn't know whether I liked the pink color of the house. Ellard replied, "Oh no, it's green." The next day, Ed and Ellard went back down to Galveston. Ellard bought the green house (it was pink inside), and Ed bought the vacant lot next door. Never did we do anything so impulsively and never did we enjoy anything so much.

Gradually Ellard got stronger, and by January 1961, was able to go back to work. That was a good year for us. Ellard was having one of the remissions characteristic of Hodgkins and felt good. In June when the children got out of school, we spent the whole month at the beach. It was a glorious time. In the mornings we woke to the sound of birds and the low roar of the ocean and looked out at the glistening sea. Each day the ocean was different. The tide came up to different levels and the color of the water changed. The color changed not only day-by-day, but sometimes several times during a day. There was a broad band of turquoise or light blue water near the shore and then further out there was the "blue water." This was a deep blue area that stretched out to the horizon. Sometimes the blue water was close into the shore, other times it was many miles out. The blue water was where the good fishing was. During the day the sea changed in response to the sky. It had dark patches where great billowing cumulus clouds were overhead. When squalls swept across it became metallic gray. Nothing could be more magnificent than the feel of the quickening wind, the sight of the rain approaching across the water, and finally the sound of the heavy subtropical rain on our shed roof. In the evenings our yard and the dunes were covered with the pastel blooms of the evening primroses, and we watched glorious sunsets across the marshes and the bay.

The whole family swam every day, walked on the beach, surf fished, crabbed, and sailed on our little sailfish. The children water-skied on the bay with Ellard piloting the motor boat, Ellard fished with men friends out on the blue water, and sometimes I went fishing far out on the ocean with him.

We made friends with the other beach dwellers and their children. The beach was virtually empty and our children ran carefree over the seagrape-covered dunes. They built forts with the neighbor children and combed the beach finding all sorts of unusual things, sometimes from the Yucatan and other distant places. They became familiar with all the small creatures in the ocean and accumulated varieties of shells. With their friends, they collected drift wood and built great piles for bonfires where we roasted gritty wieners and ate watermelon for dessert.

We were eighteen miles from the nearest store and it was just a little beach store, so we had the opportunity to teach the children about saving things and being resourceful instead of running to the store for every little thing. This was during the time of extreme concern about an atomic attack when people were building bomb shelters in their back yards, so Ellard decided it would be a good time to teach our children about survival. He declared survival week, a week in which we had to live off the land and what we could get from the sea. He permitted us to have potatoes, eggs, milk, and some produce raised on the west end of the island, but it was slim pickings. I understood why the native Indians died out on Galveston Island. For example, the land was so poor that it took an acre to provide grazing for each cow. Needless, to say we were not permitted beef. We were like The Swiss Family Robinson and we had to adapt. We ate crab and fish that I was not sure were edible and we made coquina chowder with hundreds of tiny coquinas and potatoes. It was watery and sandy, but we ate it. Somehow we made it through the week and at the end of the seven days felt very smug and hungry!

After our wonderful vacation was over, it was back to work but we spent as many weekends at the beach as possible. We arrived on the island on Friday afternoons, hoisted the flags (United States and Texas), and were in residence. We could tell what other families had arrived by their flags waving in the stiff afternoon breeze. Our Houston friends, Ed and Jackie Godwin, had now bought a house at Jamaica Beach and we and the Godwins became fast friends with a few other families who shared our love of the sea. In the mornings while the men fished, the ladies drank coffee and visited. We could watch our children from our living rooms and porches, identifying them by their respective dogs sitting patiently by their masters' towels.

The Godwins and we were especially good friends with the Hilliards, Bill and Lydia, who had preceded us at Jamaica Beach by several years. Lydia had grown up in Louisiana Bayou country and she taught me to make gumbo, delicious crab dishes, and bouillabaisse. Jackie Godwin was also a terrific cook who had lived in Tidewater, Virginia, so I learned a lot about cooking seafood from her. Frequently at night, we had potluck suppers on our porches with the Godwin children, the Hilliard children, and the Yow children listening to the parents' stories and playing under the primitive street lights, catching lightning bugs, and experiencing summer evenings much as Ellard and I had as children.

* * * * * * * *

In September, Ellard and I went to Naples where both of us gave talks. Then on to Rome, Geneva, and Basel. We had a splendid time in Europe despite the fact that Ellard was now having daily late afternoon and evening fever. He was able to enjoy mornings and afternoons until about four o'clock when he would have chills and fever and massive sweats until midnight. He was determined to have a good time, though, and to allow me to have fun. It was a wonderful experience for me socially and academically. Ellard now treated me as a peer and took every opportunity to introduce me to outstanding American and foreign infectious disease colleagues and their wives.

There was a great camaraderie in our group of Americans traveling together in Europe. Ellard was already a part of the group, but this was a first for me and I formed friendships that have lasted a lifetime with some of the greats in infectious diseases – Harry Dowling from Chicago, Maxwell Finland from Boston, Bill Kirby from Seattle, and Bill Hewitt from Los Angeles. We went to the Isle of Capri, to Pompeii, on walking tours of Rome, and on a daytrip from Geneva to Chamonix and Mont Blanc. Thirty years later, the happy memories of this trip are crystal clear and I am deeply grateful that we had this glorious time together with each other and with good friends.

* * * * * * * *

Ellard lived another five years. The story of his courage and adaptability would fill a whole book in itself. He was determined to live as normally as possible, to be as productive as possible, and to enjoy life with his family as much as possible. During those five years, he had both chronic disease and many acute life-threatening illnesses. The x-ray therapy, chemotherapy, and Hodgkins disease had destroyed his immune system, leaving him prey to terrible infections. He had long periods of severe, painful, life-threatening infections separated by periods of being able to work, write, and enjoy his children and his friends. Our extended families helped as much as possible, but they were too far away to help on a day-to-day basis. It was our friends and colleagues who rallied round and gave us tremendous support. With all their help, we were able to keep our jobs functioning, our children cared for, and our spirits bolstered most of the time.

These last years of Ellard's life were so full of living for our family – so much happiness, so much sadness. My life revolved around Ellard, but I needed to be a mother, and most of the time both parents, to the children; and I had to continue at my job. Our family life was very intense, but there was one great blessing for me. I was no longer burdened and limited by conflict. My responsibilities were very clear; I had to be three things: wife, mother, and wage-earner. It was amazing how much I could accomplish when I got rid of the drag of conflict. Looking back, I wonder how I kept so many balls in the air. It was truly a balancing act. When I leaned too far to one side on the tight rope, it was always toward Ellard. Sometimes the children got shortchanged, but my office staff helped me out in many a pinch with them, or sometimes my fellows had to assume my medical work.

* * * * * * * *

How did we manage to live so well and do so many pleasant things? We had lived very carefully until now and had a small amount of savings, intermittently Ellard's father sent generous checks, and Ellard's mother gave us some North Carolina land which we sold. Fortunately, Ellard had carried a small disability insurance policy from the time he joined the Baylor faculty. In those days, Baylor had no disability or retirement plans, and Ellard's theory was that he could afford to die but he couldn't afford to live with a long, chronic illness. It was providential that he had that foresight.

Ellard was almost a test case for Baylor disabled faculty. First, his income was cut almost in half with the reduction in his consultation practice, and then in 1962, when he was away from work for many months, his base salary was halved so now he was making a quarter of his former income. My salary was very small, but was helpful. Things were getting pretty tight, but after a year of very reduced income, a remarkable thing happened.

One evening when I was cooking supper, I had a surprising telephone call from Dr. DeBakey. As usual he was short and to the point: "Martha, I just heard about Ellard's salary being cut. I'm flying to Belgium tonight with Dr. Olson (the Dean), and by the time we get there this matter will be settled!" I barely had time to stammer my thanks and he was gone. He was as good as his word. He discussed the situation with Dr. Olson and when he returned to Houston he met with Mr. Ben Taub, and Mr. Taub offered to guarantee Ellard's full salary for life. Mr. Ben Taub had been Ellard's patient for a long time and they were very fond of each other. Also, Henry J. N. Taub and his wife, Carol, who were our age, were close friends of ours. Often Henry would come to visit Ellard after dinner and slip a check into his pajama pocket. The last year of Ellard's life, when we needed a man servant to bathe Ellard, lift him, and to drive him places, Mr. Ben sent one of his well-trained servants to live with us. One evening, Henry asked Ellard what interest rate we were paying on our beach house mortgage, and when Ellard replied seven percent, Henry was appalled. The average rate at that time was five percent. Henry bought our mortgage and reduced the interest to two percent. When Ellard died, Henry wrote off the mortgage and handed me the deed. Mr. Ben Taub and Henry J. N. Taub were so generous throughout Ellard's life and then to me and our children for many years, that I always knew I could depend on them for help if I needed it. It was a wonderful comfort to be free of serious financial concerns.

It is amazing how little Ellard's illness cost as compared to the cost of medical care today. Baylor provided medical insurance up to $100,000 for its employees. With the generosity of The Methodist Hospital and of Ellard's doctors, this lasted through numerous prolonged hospitalizations and three major operations. It gave out just a week before his death. Today, his long illness would cost at least a million dollars. Some of the difference in cost was the minimal use of intensive care facilities, the lower cost of drugs, and the lack of expensive diagnostic procedures. The latter was a mixed blessing. CAT scans, ultrasound, and magnetic resonance imaging would have greatly simplified the diagnostic procedures and would have allowed more rapid use of specific therapy. They would have saved Ellard months of suffering, brain surgery, and many other invasive procedures.

* * * * * * * *

I don't want to give the impression that I was invincible through all the heavy responsibilities and heartbreak of this period of my life. The reality is that at times I could hardly last another day. My friends were long-suffering in listening to my problems and I spent a lot of time with a psychiatrist crying, crying, crying. This was before the era of the various support groups, but I gained enough support from my friends and the psychiatrist to be able to provide support for Ellard and the children, but often I longed for escape. I had a recurrent fantasy of turning cart wheels down our long hall and out of the door.

One real escape I managed almost every year was a trip with Ina to the annual meetings of the Society for Pediatric Research and the American Pediatric Society usually held in the northeast during the first week in May. About the middle of April, Ina and I went into a flurry of activity. We went on joyful expeditions shopping for new spring suits, hats, and shoes and we prayed that no outbreak of infection would hit the newborn nursery so we could get away. My prayers were almost as fervent as those I offered up for a bicycle when I was ten years old. I remember, on the day of departure each year, riding past the hospital on the way to the airport, thinking "Please, let us get out of town before an outbreak hits the nursery." We knew that if we could get as far as the airport we wouldn't be called back. Other doctors would take over and we would make it out of town. These meetings were inspiring and tremendous fun. Ina, too, had heavy responsibilities and when we got away on our annual trip, we were like two young girls let out of school. When the plane left the ground in Houston our troubles dropped away, and when we returned they rose up to meet us but we were refreshed and ready for another stint.

The last year of Ellard's life required the most difficult balancing act that I would ever have to perform. His periods of serious illness became closer and closer together, and the periods of reprieve shorter and shorter. The children were growing up and needed my attention and my job was becoming busier. I tried to slow it down, but medicine is a jealous mistress. In the midst of this period, I began to feel like a rubber band that has been stretched too many times and is about to snap, or a piece of wire that has been bent back and forth to the breaking point. I went so far as to make diagrams to try to allocate my time better. One was a circle divided into pie slices. It always ended up with three big slices – one for Ellard, one for the children, and one for my job – and one tiny sliver for me.

In spite of increasing disability, Ellard kept trying to be active. He worked part-time, we went to the beach whenever possible, and we took two major trips. The first was another trip to Europe where we spoke in London, visited microbiologists in Copenhagen, and then went on to Prague. There Ellard gave the keynote address at an international meeting. A few hours after giving the Prague lecture, he began to have agonizing back pain and I had to get him back to Houston immediately. Leaving communist-controlled Czechoslovakia suddenly was no small feat since our passports were still in the hands of the police and because the airline on which we were traveling came to Prague only three times a week. Finally we managed to book a flight on Air India, retrieve our passports, and leave Prague before dawn the next day.

Shortly after our return, Ellard was found to have spinal cord compression from Hodgkin's and had to have back surgery. The compression led to a partial paralysis so that he could walk only with crutches and spent much of the time in a wheel chair.

Our second and last trip was to New York where Ellard was given an award by the Infectious Disease Society of America for his contributions to this field of medicine. This was a high point in his life and we celebrated it in style. Ellard's brother, who lived in New York, helped us put on a splendid party in our hotel suite, and close friends in the society made it a gala affair. Dr.

Maxwell Finland from Harvard, recognized as the dean of infectious diseases, took great pride in being the official host. It was a night to remember!

Our last big social event was a party in December 1964, when a couple of our close friends invited about twenty-five other couples to their home for a festive evening in our honor. Our children were included and had the chance to see how beloved their father was. Ellard was very frail, but no matter how sick he was, he enjoyed his friends and loved to have a good time. He told me that every day he lived he enjoyed life more and he said that he felt it was particularly important that I remain active socially so that after his death I wouldn't be so lonely and isolated.

Ellard managed to stay home for Christmas 1964 and even had Christmas presents for us. Unbeknownst to us he had shopped through the Sears catalogue. He never gave up! After Christmas, he was never able to live at home again. For several months he spent weekdays in the hospital and the weekends at home. On Saturday mornings the boys helped me bring him home and on Sunday nights we took him back.

It was a heart-breaking period for the whole family and I became more and more stressed. I rushed from one thing to another. My worst fear was that Ellard would die when I wasn't with him. His doctors and my psychiatrist tried to convince me that I couldn't be with him every minute and that I had to accept the fact that I might not be with him at the end. I knew they were right, but my anxiety was not alleviated. Many years later John told me that he felt that the tone of our lives during that time was, "Hurry, hurry, Dad's going to die!"

Looking back, I now recognize what a difficult time our children had during the last years of Ellard's illness. They didn't complain, but in recent years they have told me that our home felt like a hospital – cupboards full of bottles of intravenous fluids, needles, syringes, bandages, medicines, and the privacy of their home invaded by a succession of nurses. Ellard spent many months at home when another patient would have been in the hospital, but Bob Hettig felt that since I was a doctor, I could handle it with his coming by each night to follow Ellard's progress. We had nurses during the day and I had the night shift. We kept hospital charts for Bob to review – temperature, pulse, respiration, blood pressure, fluid intake and output, and drugs administered. All of this was a big responsibility, a drain on me, and terribly disturbing to our home life.

There was an obvious effect on Ellard, Jr., who had been popular at school and an outstanding football player; he retreated to the garage and spent all his leisure time working on a car that he built from spare parts. Catherine's grades at school dipped and she clung to home, withdrawing from friends. Later she told me that she was afraid to leave home, because when she came home her dad might be dead. John showed less effect during this time, but subsequently I learned how difficult it had been growing up without an able-bodied father and without one with whom he could have the father-son disagreements so necessary to teen age boys (how could he argue with a seriously ill father?).

Throughout all of this, I remember few vocal complaints about their father's illness, but one eruption was very telling. One day when the family couldn't do something that was important to Ellard, Jr., he burst out (to John, Catherine and me – not in his father's hearing), "Cancer, Cancer, Cancer. It's an excuse for everything that anybody doesn't want to do!" (Reflecting on all of this and observing other families in similar situations, there is no doubt in my mind that long, severe illness in the home is disruptive to all the family members.)

I remember the winter of 1965 as being gray, rainy, and gloomy. My days consisted of going to the hospital each morning to see how Ellard was, then to work, home for dinner with the children, and back to the hospital to spend the evening with Ellard. For several months he had been home on weekends, but by spring, he was in the hospital full time. He got very tired of being shut in, so in early March, when our friend Henry J.N. Taub asked what he could do for Ellard, I suggested that he arrange for an ambulance to take Ellard to the beach house. The children were on spring break, so the whole family plus a wonderful nurse went to the beach for a week. Ellard spent most of the time in his bed by the window looking out at the sky, the sea, and the children on the beach. In the evenings, we lifted him into a big chair in the living room for cocktail hour and dinner. The cortisone he was receiving gave him a good appetite, so I cooked special meals. He commented that he couldn't have better food at Antoine's in New Orleans. It was a good week and valuable to all of us.

After that, Ellard had no more weekends at home, but one of the children or I spent Saturday and Sunday evenings with him – bringing in a special dinner and eating with him, reading to him, or sharing TV programs. He and I spent long, loving evenings together. By April, we were both aware that he had very little time left. Now he was in an oxygen tent – this was before the use of intranasal tubes to deliver oxygen. With his usual adaptability, he read the paper in the tent, reviewed cases for other doctors, and worked on plans for enlarging the beach house.

Even this late in his life, Ellard still had a strong sense of responsibility and a great sense of humor. About a month before he died, we received a notice that we were being investigated by the Internal Revenue Service, and I thought that I would, of course, have to handle it. But Ellard said, "No, you won't be able to justify some of my business expenses. We will have the IRS agent meet with us and our accountant here in my hospital room." So we set up a card table and chair for the agent, our accountant came, and we were ready. When the agent arrived and saw this terribly ill man in the oxygen tent, he was visibly shaken and stammered out, "Your return is being questioned because we don't understand how two doctors could make so little." So we proceeded to show him how. Each of us had compulsive secretaries who kept detailed records, and we began to walk him laboriously through them. In a very few minutes, he said, "That's enough – I don't need to see anymore." Our accountant and I escorted the pale T-man to the elevator where as he escaped into it, he said, "Good-bye, being in a hospital makes me sick." A week later, we received a seventeen dollar refund from the IRS. Ellard and I laughed heartily about that great coup. I have never been investigated again, but if I should be, I have a plan. I'll put on a little lace cap like the wolf playing grandmother in "Little Red Riding Hood," and jump into an oxygen tent for the interview.

Late in March 1965, Ellard asked for his mother and brother to come to see him (his Dad, my wonderful friend, had died at Christmas). After their visit he told me that now he wanted to be only with the children and me. He discussed plans for the children with me and made three suggestions to me – "Don't get married again for a year, don't change jobs for a year, and don't sell the house for a year." He said he had seen many widows become frantic and make bad decisions in the first year after their husbands died.

About ten days before his death, he asked me to put the beach house plans away. That was a signal to me that he was dying. A few days later he told me that he was very tired and ready to go. He extracted a pledge from me, Bob Hettig, and Ed Ory that there would be no heroic efforts to prolong his life – no tubes, no machines. In April, on Easter morning, he lapsed into a coma and in three days he was gone. He had a death of quiet dignity. Never was there any greater outpouring of love than that extended to us. Ellard's colleagues had made sure that, before his death, he was honored in every way possible. I like to think that his forty-seven years were as full as many peoples' three score and ten. And when he died in 1965, I felt as if he had had a rich and victorious life.

* * * * * * * *

I thought that I had grieved so much during his long illness that I wouldn't have to grieve very long after his death. I was completely wrong. I hadn't begun to grieve. My anguish was terrible. We had been so close that I felt as if half of me was gone. And there was a terrible visceral feeling as if I had a deep stab wound in my abdomen that wouldn't heal from the inside but was just covered on the surface by a thin layer of skin. I wanted to lie down and beat my breast, and if it hadn't been for my children, I would have wanted to die. I didn't know there could be such pain. I needed to stay home with my children for a while and grieve, but Dr. Blattner insisted that I would be better off working. So the children went back to school and I continued to work harder than ever. We had practiced stiff-upper-lip for so long that we didn't know any other way to live.

The children and I spent a lot of time together that summer after Ellard's death but we didn't go to the beach. I don't know how they felt, but I couldn't go that year without Ellard. The house remained boarded up. Before his death, Ellard had given me some money to give to Ellard, Jr., when he graduated from high school. He wanted young Ellard to have the opportunity to go to Europe with some of his friends and suggested that Catherine, John, and I join him for the last three weeks of his sojourn. So all summer, we had that to plan and look forward to. In August, Catherine, John, and I met young Ellard in London. We planned to go to Glasgow where I had been invited to speak and then on to Paris, Rome, and Switzerland.

We never went to Glasgow. In London, when I didn't have a work schedule to meet, I fell apart. The realization of our loss of Ellard hit me full blast and I was physically sick. It was impossible for me to go on a speaking trip, so I had to cancel that part of the trip and just spend time with the family. During the daytime I was fine. We went sight seeing and took lengthy walking tours each place we went, but at night, I had the severe insomnia described by so many people who have lost family members. I must have read a paperback book per night. In Rome, Cathy experienced the same kind of falling apart that I had in London, and told me how terribly she missed her father. The trip was not only uninterrupted family time, but also served to start our real grieving and as a beginning of the long healing process.

In the fall, young Ellard was off to college. Our family was shrinking, and now John was in an all female milieu after having lived his first fourteen years in a male-dominated home. He was quite verbal about it, but despite his complaints, we had a pretty good time together. He had lots of good friends and our family room seemed always to be full of boys talking and John's jazz band, The Mixed Nuts, playing jazz at thousands of decibels.

It was a good thing that I remembered Ellard's injunction about not remarrying right away. The year after his death, I was almost frenetic socially. I sorely missed my role as a wife, and I wanted a companion of my own age. It was a matter of loss of closeness, not a matter of no social life. Fortunately, our social life had really never waned, so our friends included me in social activities. Bob Hettig escorted me to medical school functions and to all the parties of the couples with whom Ellard and I had been friends. Bob had the same circle of friends, so it was all very easy and natural. But it wasn't like having a real partner.

After a while, I began to go out with other eligible men.

Courtship after forty was a unique experience, especially with teenage children monitoring it. It was especially unusual when young Ellard was home from college in the summer. He kept me on a tight rein. When the men came to call, he let them in and looked them over. He would whisper things to me like, "You've got to be kidding!" and when my escort brought me home at the end of the evening, the bright porch light would flash on and Ellard would open the door and say, "All right, it's midnight, Mother; you'd better come in." Bob Hettig said that it took real courage to run the gamut of my children in order to take me out.

I was pretty inept at courtship, and the men seemed equally out of practice. In spite of this, one or two were courting me with obvious serious intent, but we weren't right for each other, and I was scuttling backwards like a crawfish. However, I was looking for someone with whom I could start over and I was certainly the most vulnerable the first year after Ellard's death, so I could have rushed in to an unsuitable marriage. It was a good thing that I had my children's appraisals to make me take a more sanguine attitude.

I finally settled down and invested more in activities with my children. After a year I felt able to go back down to the beach house, and then worked with a builder in enlarging it as Ellard and I had planned. It was a grand project for the family, and the beach house turned out to be a great thing for all of us.

Despite all this activity and working hard at my job, after two years I was still grieving and depressed. Each morning when I got up I was depressed, at work I was all right, and then as I started home, the cloud came down over me again. The nearer I got to the house the worse it got. Finally, I realized that the house had too many sad memories for me, and I began to consider moving. Since the maintenance of a house and the grounds was burdensome, I opted for a high-rise apartment near John's and Catherine's school and discussed this possibility with them. They agreed that it would be all right with them. From the day we moved in to that spacious bright apartment with its fantastic view of the Houston skyline, I felt normal again. One of my friends told me that it was time for me to stop being a sad widow and to start being a merry widow. I took the advice. At last I was able to really enjoy life again.

Chapter 12

The Congenital Rubella Epidemic and Inching up the Academic Ladder

JUST WHEN I WAS THE busiest at home, the last six months of Ellard's life, I had to meet the challenge of another major epidemic. In October 1964, an infant was born at J.D. with enlargement of the liver and spleen and a strange, purplish rash. Ina and Dr. Jack Rudolph, a member of her newborn section at J.D., thought that these abnormalities might be due to some intrauterine infection, possibly congenital syphilis, but the diagnosis of syphilis did not prove to be true. Shortly thereafter, another child was born with similar findings, and although the patient did not fit the usual picture of congenital rubella (which up until then had been thought to be limited to microcephaly, heart disease, and cataracts), specimens were sent to Dr. Melnick's virology lab where rubella was isolated. Now the diagnosis of congenital rubella (an intrauterine infection of the infant resulting from the mother's having German measles or "three-day measles" during pregnancy) was established. It was certainly not surprising that we were seeing congenital rubella in the fall of 1964, since there had been a nationwide epidemic of rubella in young women in the winter and spring, just nine months before.

During November, more and more rubella-infected infants

with various combinations of poor growth, microcephaly, cataracts, heart disease, and the newly recognized features of liver and spleen enlargement and rash were born, not only at J.D., but all over Houston, Texas, and the nation. It rapidly became clear that we had to make some special arrangements for these very sick infants.

Early in December I went to see Ina at her home where she was convalescing from a surgical procedure. We discussed the situation over cups of tea, Ina's Scottish approach to all problems. We agreed that we needed special facilities and an organized team to diagnose the children, to provide care, and to study the problems of congenital rubella. Immediately, each of us declared that she could not possibly handle such a big undertaking at the moment. Nonetheless, we began to plan and to make lists of people who were needed to study these children who had disease involving so many systems. Both of us loved to make organizational charts and soon we were hooked. In an hour or two, we agreed that we had to form a Baylor Cooperative Study Group. Ina said she would feel better soon and in the meantime her section at J.D. would, of course, work with me; but it was up to me to get the project started and I was dispatched to interview potential team members.

The rubella experience was a classical example of serendipity. Everything was in place to enable us to detect and treat infants with rubella and to learn about the new features they were presenting. Ina and the members of her neonatology section were in the position to detect the infants, Dr. Melnick's lab was experienced in isolating the virus (a technique that had been available only two years), Texas Children's Hospital had just opened a federally supported clinical research unit in which the children could be evaluated in depth at no expense to the families, and I had an infectious disease fellow who could devote full time to this problem.

Recruiting an expert team proved to be no problem. All the individuals I interviewed were enthusiastic and agreed to participate in the program for an extended period. Ina, Joe Melnick, and I would coordinate the effort and the team would consist of about eighteen members, including neonatologists, cardiologists, ophthalmologists, neurologists, radiologists, otolaryngolo gists, radiologists, pathologists, virologists, and many others. All of these specialists were needed since rubella affected so many parts of the body.

The Clinical Research Center was a great boon to us as clinicians, but an even greater boon to the families. These were terribly ill children born to mostly young mothers. The majority of the infants were first children. The shock and grief of their children's problems was devastating to these young couples and it was fortunate that we could help them. The physicians on the rubella team donated their services, the Clinical Research Center provided the expensive diagnostic procedures and care that were necessary during the first few weeks of life. Most of the babies with rubella were born to young families who could not afford the medical expenses, even with the help of the grandparents.

Where would we get the money to handle such a massive medical catastrophe? Again Ina and I drank tea and planned. I would ask the NIH whether I could use the funds from the diarrhea grant for rubella research, and Ina would request that the Hartford Foundation let her change the focus of her study, "The Neurologic Development of the infant," to the study of rubella. Both institutions agreed promptly. Joe Melnick said he had funds to finance the necessary virologic studies. Still we needed money for many things – transportation of the infants between hospitals, research nurses, secretarial assistance, social workers. At first, Ina sometimes paid for the transportation of the infants by ambulance out of her own pocket.

The Department of Pediatrics had no funds to help us, but Dr. Blattner contacted Mrs. Lenore Hamman, a wealthy Houstonian who had a twenty-year-old son damaged by congenital rubella. She agreed to have lunch with Ina and me. Remarkable things happened during that luncheon meeting. Mrs. Hamman offered us fifteen thousand dollars to begin the rubella program and equally as important, she gave us valuable information about the course of congenital rubella. Since Ina and I were both parents, we realized that parents often observe things that doctors miss, so we listened attentively. Mrs Hamman told us that, despite the dogma that rubella babies were born with static fixed problems, this was not true. She had observed that her son's problems changed with time, especially the neurologic aspects and the degree of his deafness. Doctors had always believed that all of the damage from congenital rubella occurred in the first trimester of pregnancy and there was no further progression of the disease thereafter.

Mrs Hamman was right. In 1963, Dr. Charles Alford, working with Dr. Thomas Weller at Harvard, found that the virus remained in the fetus up to at least five months of gestation. Soon we and others were to find that the virus was still present in the infant at birth, and in some infants for over a year. It was capable of causing continuing damage. Listening to Mrs Hamman alerted Ina to the potential for progression of the disease. Ina's observations of this progression led her to write an article describing congenital rubella as a dynamic, changing disease.

Mrs Hamman was a generous person. She asked me to come out to her home that very afternoon to pick up the check. When I looked at it, the amount was for more than fifteen thousand dollars. She commented, "You may need more than you think." Again she was right. We were to write numerous grant requests over a good many years.

Ina and I were ideal collaborators. I was particularly good at acute care, and she was good not only at acute management, but also had the staying power to provide long-term care. My role, with the help of my fellow, was to coordinate the early evaluation and care of the infants, and to collect and transport appropriate specimens for virologic study. Her role, with the assistance of her section members, was to detect the sick infants, transfer them to the Clinical Research Center, and provide the subsequent long-term care.

We soon discovered the magnitude of this project. These infants required constant care for a multitude of problems. Early in their lives, bleeding was a major problem, as was heart failure. Many had open heart surgery in the first few months of life to correct congenital defects. At about four months of age, eye surgery was performed to remove cataracts. Many infants had prolonged liver disease; others were severely damaged neurologically – some with cerebral palsy or seizures. In some, deafness was apparent early; in others it was detected later. These children encountered one problem after another.

One of the worst problems was that the infants continued to have virus in their throat, urine, and spinal fluid for about a year, so that they were contagious and were a threat to women of childbearing age. This meant that when the infants were well enough to go home from the hospital, the parents could not take them out to church, the grocery store, or to any place where they might transmit the virus. Many infants were so sick that they had to remain hospitalized. Those whose parents could afford it were cared for in special isolation in private hospitals. For others, whose parents were indigent, a special rubella ward had to be created at J.D.

By three months into the Houston epidemic, we had worked with twenty-five rubella babies. We were now familiar with what Dr. Blattner termed the "expanded rubella syndrome." It was time for us to publish our early findings. On a rainy Saturday morning, Dr. Blattner, Ina, Jack Rudolph, and I met to summarize the data. Never had I invested myself so deeply in any project and I desperately wanted to be the senior author on this first paper describing the expanded syndrome, but it had to be written immediately and Ellard was too ill for me to undertake it. Dr. Blattner suggested that since he, Ina, and I were too busy, that Jack Rudolph write it. I had always thought I was a big enough person and a sufficiently dedicated scientist to remember that the important thing is the contribution of new knowledge, not who gets the credit. This time, however, I was not so generous in spirit and was bitterly disappointed that I was unable to write the report. This was an occasion when I had a difficult time balancing my priorities. In March, the *Journal of the American Medical Association* published this first paper on the expanded rubella syndrome (Rudolph et al. 1965).

But I felt better when Dr. Saul Krugman of New York University invited me to speak at a rubella symposium. I accepted the invitation although I didn't know whether I would be able to attend (if I couldn't, someone else on our team could take my place). Ten days after Ellard's death, I forced myself to go to Washington where I presented the Houston experience with rubella–I remember it vividly because I was feeling terrible and gave a poor presentation. Probably I should not have tried to go. I should have been at home with my children, but it meant a great deal to me to be a part of that conference. It was an affirmation (for me) that I had made a contribution to solving the rubella problem, and thereafter I was invited to the national workshops where vaccine development and control measures were discussed.

Throughout 1965, infants with congenital rubella continued to be born in large numbers all over the United States. With their deafness and blindness, I felt as if we were seeing large numbers of Helen Kellers, but these babies had the added disadvantage of never having seen or heard, whereas Helen Keller had sight and hearing until she was about two years old. In this epidemic in 1964, there were 11,000 fetal deaths and 20,000 infants born with defects due to rubella. The epidemic caused tremendous suffering and cost the nation's economy an estimated two billion dollars.

I worked in the congenital rubella program for two years. Then Dr. John Montgomery, a member of the infectious disease section, coordinated the rubella follow-up clinic for three years. Ina, with her remarkable tenacity and perseverance, continued to raise funds and follow the lives of these children for eighteen years. She and John Montgomery did a remarkable job of using multiple community resources, such as the cerebral palsy center, the Lighthouse for The Blind, The School for Speech and Hearing, and the local March of Dimes organization. This was truly a wonderful example of an all-out community effort.

Why am I telling so much about the rubella epidemic? First, because it was the most satisfying clinical research of my career. It was a unique situation in which we were in a position to give all these children optimal care, rich and poor alike. And we, with other investigators around the country, were able to define the problem clearly, so that within five years, a vaccine was available to prevent this terrible illness. Today congenital rubella occurs in about 10 or fewer children per year and the cases usually occur in religious groups who refuse immunization. The rubella story is one of cooperation between physicians and scientists all over the nation that led to the conquering of a devastating problem. It is truly a story of a medical triumph!

The second reason I am writing so much about rubella is that working with rubella influenced the course of all my subsequent clinical investigations. I continued to work with infectious diseases in children of all ages, but now my research became focused on the prevention of perinatal infections; that is, infection of the infant while in the uterus, during the process of birth, or in the first few weeks after birth.

* * * * * * * *

Now I entered a happy, productive period of my life. For the first time I was free of heavy domestic responsibilities. Ellard was in college, John and Catherine were in high school, and we had a young housekeeper who shouldered all the household duties and was a wonderful companion for John and Cathy. Once again we began to have fun at home and at the beach. I enjoyed John's and Cathy's friends and they enjoyed mine. We had dinner parties in town and house parties at the beach.

There were opportunities to entertain fascinating people – famous people in medicine and in music. Some of these were people I knew, others were asked to contact me by friends in other cities. Many were from the United States, others were from abroad. I once read that famous people are often lonely when they travel. People either entertain them at large, meaningless cocktail parties or receptions or they are afraid to approach a celebrity and don't ask them out at all. As a result, the famous spend solitary evenings in hotels. With this in mind, when they called, I asked them to visit in our home. They sounded eager to have a family dinner with us and spend a quiet evening in our home. John and Catherine were both involved in music so they were very thrilled when Conductor Charles Munch came to dinner. Also Sir John and Lady Barbarolli contacted us when they moved to Houston where he was to be the conductor of the Houston Symphony Orchestra. They spent time with us and then Sir John invited us to a Saturday morning rehearsal of the Symphony. Timidly we entered the back door of the symphony hall, walked through a sort of subterranean passage and then up to the auditorium where we slipped quietly into seats. Sir John spied us and waved us up onto the stage. He told us that to really experience the rehearsal, we had to sit "under his baton," so John sat in the brass section, Cathy with the violins, and I with the cellos. What a thrilling experience!

* * * * * * * *

Things were equally good at work. I was inching up the academic ladder. In 1965, after I was in a position to work full time, I had been promoted to the rank of associate professor. It had taken me two years as an instructor and eight years as an assistant professor to advance to associate professor. This was five years longer than my peers, but I felt that it was fair because there had been so many periods when I couldn't work full time.

I felt good about my progress in pediatrics and loved working with children. Each of them was unique and it was fun to get to know them. I especially enjoyed relating to children who were about four to twelve years old. They were old enough so you could reason with them, but they were still fresh and innocent and said such unexpected things. One day I said to a little boy, "I bet you are seven years old." He asked, "How can you tell?" " Well," I answered, "I looked at your teeth." Without a moment's hesitation he countered, "Let me look at your teeth so that I can tell how old you are." I must not have evidenced this enjoyment to my own children, though, because once when a person remarked to my twelve-year-old daughter, Catherine, "Your mother is a pediatrician, so she must love children," Catherine's dry answer was, "No, she likes germs."

And I did like working with germs. Although I had entered the field of infectious diseases by chance, there could not have been a more perfect choice for me. I loved the excitement of determining the cause of a child's illness, the certainty with which infectious diseases could be diagnosed (often seeing the causative organism under the microscope), the availability of specific treatment for most infections, and the gratification of curing patients quickly. Children have such remarkable ability to recover that they respond to treatment much more rapidly than adults. Of course, there were sad instances when we couldn't help patients, but that was not the rule in infectious diseases after antibiotics became available.

The practice of infectious diseases was never dull. Not a week passed that I didn't see a disease I had never seen before or some unusual variation of a common disease. I think that being an infectious disease specialist is like being a detective and requires hound-dog tenacity. My fellows and I were frequently involved in cases that required intensive investigation of a child's environment, and rarely did a year go by when we were not busy dealing with outbreaks or epidemics of infection in our teaching hospitals, other Houston hospitals, or in the Houston community.

I was gaining a tremendous amount of clinical experience and having a wonderful time interacting with students, residents, and fellows. There was only one problem. I was drowning in work. Houston was growing rapidly, and the number of children with infectious disease problems was keeping pace. It was clear that a lone faculty member could not see them all, teach, and carry on research. So somehow, I had to find ways to add faculty members to the "Infectious Disease Section." My situation was not unique. All of the section heads in the department of pediatrics had the same problem. All of us needed more faculty members.

The department was growing rapidly, and Dr. Blattner was building one of the most comprehensive pediatric programs in the nation. We now had numerous subspecialty sections including cardiology, hematology, endocrinology, neurology, and neonatology. All of the sections were headed by vigorous, well-trained, ambitious young doctors. To me, it was like pioneering on a big ranch with each of us developing our own area and I, like all the other section heads, had to come up with the necessary resources to support my program. I felt more confident, because I had been promoted to full professor. I continued to have a vision of building a section composed of faculty members, each with a special area of expertise in infectious diseases (bacterial infections, viral infections, immunologic problems), so that we could provide state-of-the-art care for our patients and so that we could add new knowledge to the field. I had to develop my own "back forty."

I had observed Dr. Blattner's technique in building the department and would use the same strategy in building my section. He selected promising residents, advised them to go away for subspecialty training and brought them back as members of the faculty. I selected outstanding residents to spend time in fellowship training with me, encouraged them to acquire additional skills either at other schools or in the basic science departments at Baylor, and promised them that I would try to provide faculty positions at the completion of their training.

In 1966, Dr. Blattner permitted me to add two faculty members, Dr. Mary Ann South and Dr. John Montgomery (Jack) to the infectious disease section. Both of them were expert in immunology (but in different aspects). In rapid succession during the next few years, we added Dr. Larry Taber and Dr. Fred Barrett. Larry's expertise was in virology and Fred's interests were bacteriology and epidemiology. All four of them, Mary Ann, Jack, Larry, and Fred, helped obtain their financial support. Mary Ann applied for and received a research career development award from the NIH. Jack became the coordinator for the rubella clinic, Larry was the director of the pediatric outpatient department at Ben Taub Hospital, and Fred was the first infections control officer at Texas Children's Hospital. The five of us were equally resourceful about funding our research, much of which had to be done at night and on weekends.

Together we raised funds to establish an infectious disease laboratory at Texas Children's Hospital and added a sixth faculty member, Dr. Ed Mason, a microbiologist, to supervise the lab. Now my dream had become a reality. We had a comprehensive infectious disease group that could provide optimal care to patients and attract fellows not only from the Baylor residency program, but from schools all around the country.

It was stimulating to be surrounded by well-trained people with inquiring minds. Research projects were dreamed up around my dining room table in Houston and sitting around the fireplace at the beach house on cold, foggy winter nights. The infectious disease faculty spent lots of time together – consulting on difficult cases, discussing new ideas, traveling to meetings, entertaining visiting professors in Houston, writing papers at the beach, and just plain having a good time. Our fellows shared in the camaraderie. The faculty and fellows were truly an extended family for me and for John and Cathy. Once I asked Larry whether he felt like my son. He replied "No, I feel like your younger brother." Mary Ann lived in the same apartment house that the children and I did, and we spent a lot of time together. It was not unusual for Mary Ann and me to get into impassioned discussions about the possible functions of T lymphocytes (the cells now involved in AIDS) and other fascinating matters. These discussions often went on long after midnight.

One of the greatest things about the members of our section was that we all shared the same idealism about dealing with patients and their families. As section head, it was wonderful for me to know that no matter who was on call, the patients would not only have expert medical care, but they and their families would also be treated compassionately.

I had many good years working at Baylor, but for me, the years that Mary Ann, Jack, Fred, Larry, Ed and I were together were the golden era of the infectious disease section. I was so happy developing my own back forty, that friends from other schools would say, "For goodness sakes, don't ask Martha anything about her section, because you won't be able to get her to stop talking."

Chapter 13

A Time of Transition

In 1970, my children were away at college and things were going so well in our expanded infectious disease section that I decided it was a good time for me to get some additional training. Ever since I had worked with rubella, I had wanted to work with another congenital viral infection, cytomegalovirus infection (usually referred to as CMV), that causes severe handicaps including mental retardation, deafness, blindness, and cerebral palsy. I wanted to learn about CMV infection in women of childbearing age so I could search for possible methods to prevent infection in pregnant women and the transmission of infection to their infants.

To do this, I needed to understand the virus itself, which would require studying under the direction of an expert. The best place to study was at the Harvard School of Public Health in the laboratory of Dr. Thomas Weller. Dr. Weller was one of the first persons to grow CMV and was a leader in the field. He was also a major contributor to the knowledge of congenital rubella and had been awarded the Nobel prize for his work with poliovirus, work that made the development of the polio vaccine possible.

I went to ask Dr. Blattner whether I could go on sabbatical

leave for a year. He agreed, so I wrote to Dr. Weller. To my great delight, Dr. Weller responded promptly saying that he could offer me supervision, bench space, and a technician if I would interview and examine patients with CMV infection. This was a fantastic opportunity, so I made arrangements for my Baylor work to be continued, made plans to close my apartment and bought heavy winter clothes for the Boston winter. When all was set, I went to report my progress to Dr. Blattner. He surprised me by saying, "Well, you'll have to go see the dean." Happily, I went off to see the dean, a Harvard Medical School graduate, thinking that he would be impressed by a faculty member's having such a splendid opportunity to study at his alma mater. Instead, he asked, "Who is going to pay your salary?" I replied that since I was eligible for a sabbatical, I had assumed that the school would do so. He quickly dispelled that misconception saying, "Oh no, your chairman has to pay you." That was the kiss of death. Of course, Dr. Blattner had no funds for this purpose, so bitterly disappointed, I had to write Dr. Weller telling him that I couldn't come. This was not a matter of discrimination against me. Subsequently, I learned that Baylor was noted for giving few sabbaticals. In fact, it became a Baylor joke that if you were allowed a sabbatical it was usually a "terminal sabbatical," a way of easing you out.

Looking back, it was shortsighted of the school, and of me, not to work out some way to take advantage of this great opportunity. It would have put me in the position to get a large grant for the study of CMV at Baylor. Many times since, I have wondered why I didn't borrow the money and go to Boston, but then I remember that I had three children in college and that it was out of the question.

About this time, money for our family became a serious issue. Since Ellard's death we had been living on my salary and Ellard's life insurance. Now the insurance was running out and it became clear that I had to be more realistic about money. Doctors, other than surgeons, in academic medicine, almost never make as much as doctors in private practice, but they accept that as a given fact when they decide on an academic career. Now, however, I was making less than half of what practicing pediatricians in Houston were making and I suspected that I was making less than the male professors in the Department of Pediatrics. They couldn't be living as well as they were and be educating their children if they were not making more than I was. I tried to find out the salary range for the professors in our department, but neither Dr. Blattner nor the business manager would divulge that information. I knew that Ina was making about what I was, maybe a little more because she had more seniority, but it was impossible to find out what the range was for the men. Fortunately, just at this time, the overall business arrangements of the department were changed, and I learned that some of the male associate professors were making more than I was as a full professor. This was grossly unfair and I knew that I had to be assertive about the situation.

The first thing I did was to consult Bill Daeschner, who was now Chairman of the Department of Pediatrics at the University of Texas medical school in Galveston, to ask him about salary ranges at the University of Texas medical schools. He steered me to a publication that contained the range of salaries in all five of these state schools. By this standard, my salary was shockingly out of line. I was making about two-thirds of the norm. This was clearly a case of sexual discrimination and I had to do something about it. I had always hated talking about money and often ended up holding the short end of the stick. When I was in college, my mother had been concerned about this and said to me, "Well, I give up on trying to convince you, but when you have to have the money, you'll stand up for yourself." She was right. Now I had to have more self interest.

This was an opportune time to try to get the matter straightened out. In 1970, the Women's Equity Action League had filed a complaint with the U.S. Department of Labor demanding a review of all colleges and universities that received federal money, to investigate their compliance with antidiscriminatory regulations. In that year, more than 160 of these institutions were brought into court. I was not aware of these facts when I went to see Dr. Blattner about my salary, but I knew that if he did not agree to a substantial increase, I could go to the Baylor Grievance Committee and file a complaint. Dr. Blattner and I had a violent argument during which he assumed a parental role and tried to make me feel like an ungrateful child. I was having none of it. I told him that we had to get the matter settled or I would go to the Grievance Committee for arbitration. He finally agreed to give me an 18% raise over a period of two years. I should have insisted on a 33% raise, but I decided to settle for the smaller amount and to think about changing jobs. Things were never really good between Dr. Blattner and me again. It was a sad rift, but he was of his generation who thought it was all right to underpay women, and I was of my generation who knew it was wrong.

Sometime in the early seventies, a woman professor at Baylor organized a class action suit against the school for underpaying women, but I declined to join. The suit was won and although I had not participated, I was offered $10,000. I refused the money because Baylor was like a second home to me and I didn't want to sue the school that Ellard and I had helped to build. At Baylor, except for my salary, I had always been given equal opportunity and I felt that I should have spoken up sooner or should have left Baylor if I knew that I wasn't being paid fairly. I preferred to have a good relationship with the school than to have the $10,000, and in the long run, that attitude paid off. I am not recommending the course of action that I took; it was just best for me.

The feminist movement had other effects on my career. Now a number of outstanding opportunities were open to women who had the training and experience to accept them, so I reaped the rewards of the movement although I had never been involved in women's liberation. I had resisted participating in it partly because of its stridency and partly because I was too busy trying to live as a liberated woman to have time to talk about it. All of the time I had been in medicine, beginning in my medical school days, I had tried to dispel the image of a woman doctor's being unfeminine. I wanted to show that a woman could be a competent doctor without acting masculine. It was impossible for me to suddenly become militant.

However, many years later, after reading about the long fight for women's rights beginning in the nineteenth century, I realized that many of the women who affected important changes were not militant and I understood why really strong positions were necessary to achieve the status women have today.

I owe a personal debt of gratitude to the women who waged the battles and those who continue to do so (Rosenberg 1992).

The early 1970s were the years of token women and token blacks, and there were many times when I felt that I had unusual opportunities because I was the token woman, but I also like to think that I had earned many of the opportunities by hard work and ability.

Nineteen-seventy also signaled the beginning of a marked increase in the number of women entering the medical profession. In the first part of the decade, the number of women who enrolled in medical school increased four-fold, and this trend continued. A report from the American Medical Association shows that between 1970 and 1990, the percentage of women entering medical school rose from 9.4% to 40.2% (AMA 1991). There was, of course, a lag in the number of women who were ready for leadership positions, so that those who had the requisite training and experience found themselves in an enviable position.

Still it came as a surprise to me when I was asked to serve on the Infectious Diseases Committee of the American Academy of Pediatrics, an organization of 50,000 pediatricians. This committee is made up of members from nine districts in the United States. I was the member appointed from the seventh district (Alabama, Louisiana, and Texas). The committees provides an invaluable service to pediatricians of the United States, Canada, and South and Central America. It meets two or three times a year to formulate guidelines for the diagnosis, treatment, and prevention of infectious diseases and to update The Redbook, the bible of infectious diseases for pediatricians. Working on this committee was a tremendous educational experience and an opportunity to form warm friendships with colleagues from other areas and institutions. I served as a member of the committee for eight years and was chairman during the last two. As chairman, I was invited to speak throughout the U.S., in Canada, and in Central and South America. In addition, the chairman served as a liaison member of other national policy-making committees. This job with the Academy provided insight into the workings of medicine in our country.

My appointment in the early seventies to another national

committee, The Board of Scientific Counselors at the National Institutes of Health (NIH), provided another educational opportunity. On this committee, I learned about the research activities of the NIH at the Bethesda campus and at NIH laboratories based in Montana, Panama, Atlanta, and Hawaii. This experience also afforded the opportunity to learn about the interaction between the NIH and the Centers for Disease Control (CDC) in Atlanta. This committee assignment was for three years and again, perhaps as the token woman, I was the chairman during the last year.

Working on these two national committees was an enriching experience and opened my eyes to many career opportunities as I began to think seriously about changing jobs. I had been at Baylor about twenty years, a long time for an academician to stay at one medical school and I felt the need for a change.

However, I didn't pursue the matter of changing jobs right away because my personal life in Houston was too absorbing. After the Harvard sabbatical fell through, I decided to build the contemporary house Ellard and I had always planned, and the combination of my work, meeting with the architect and builder, and scratching together the money to pay for the house filled much of my time. The rest was filled with family affairs – Catherine and young Ellard both got married and Catherine presented me with my first grandchild, Megan, the joy of my life.

Then things began to pall. It was terribly hard to get money to keep research going. Money was tight in the early seventies at all the granting agencies, and those of us trying to pursue clinical research had to rely heavily on local support. Fortunately, Houston was still relatively prosperous and Houstonians were generous but, unfortunately, neither Ina nor I was doing very glamorous research. The bulk of donations went to cardiovascular or cancer research, so Ina and I wrote grant after grant and survived from year to year on donations from individuals in Houston. On two occasions, women I happened to meet in Jamail's, Houston's gourmet grocery store, asked about my research and offered financial support. On one of these occasions, I was given a donation that paid a fellow's salary for a year. The women of Houston were supportive of both Ina and me, but it is hard for individuals or small foundations to provide the substantial, ongoing support needed to keep a research program functioning.

To keep our spirits up, Ina and I had a number of quotations and slogans to bolster each other's morale when we received long-awaited letters from granting agencies, only to learn that our requests had been rejected. Our favorite was, "There's a dance in the old dame yet," a quotation from Don Marquis' characters, archy and mehitabel (Marquis 1927). The story of mehitabel, an old but gutsy alley cat who is on her ninth life, is told by archy, a cockroach who types poems on a newsroom typewriter, but can't press the keys for capital letters or for punctuation. No matter what trouble befalls mehitabel or what scrapes she gets into, she always sings some variation of her favorite song,

> my youth i shall never forget
> but there s nothing i really regret
> *wotthehell wotthehell*
> there s a dance in the old dame yet
> *toujours gai toujours gai*

At times Ina and I felt so desperate for funds, that we joked about dressing as men, putting nylon stockings over our heads, and robbing a bank. Who would ever suspect two Baylor women doctors? I fantasized that we would be called the Mutt and Jeff robbers – I was tall and Ina was short. At times, we used our own money to keep going and keep going we did, but I began to think that I had better move to a different school where, at least initially, a budget would be supplied.

Finally, I felt so discouraged that I went to Galveston to discuss my career situation with Bill Daeschner, my ever-present, reliable ally. He volunteered to put out the word I was interested in changing jobs. Meanwhile, I decided I had to do something to revive my spirits more quickly – and I did something very extravagant. I thought, "I've spent all this money sending my children to camp, now I'm going to spend something on myself – I'm going to a spa." So off I went to the Greenhouse, the luxurious spa between Dallas and Fort Worth.

What a week! When the sophisticated, manicured woman

manager asked me what I wanted to achieve during the week, I said I wanted to lose five pounds and wanted to be protected from the telephone. I didn't want to receive a single phone call – that week was a period of real change. I had a wonderful time with the other women there and felt like a sorority girl. We laughed, suffered together on our starvation diets, groaned about our aching muscles from the enforced exercise, and shared stories about why we were at the Greenhouse. Some were trying to get over divorces or sad love affairs. Others, like me, were trying to escape from responsibility for a bit. One attractive, but plump, young woman from Georgia was there to lose weight and improve her appearance before going with her husband on a campaign tour for a candidate who was seeking the democratic presidential nomination. She told us his name was Jimmy Carter. The others of us thought, "Yeah, yeah, we've never heard of him. He hasn't got a chance."

I rested, exercised, and dieted, was massaged, manicured, pedicured, given a new hair style and taught to put on makeup properly. At the end of the week, we were escorted to Neiman Marcus where I bought elegant clothes to wear on job interviews. When I arrived back in Houston, trim and rested, I felt like a movie star.

Now I began to look seriously at positions at other medical schools. First, I went to Philadelphia to be interviewed for the position of Chairman of the Department of Pediatrics at the University of Pennsylvania and Physician-in-Chief of the Philadelphia Children's Hospital. My principal interviewer was Dr. Everett Koop, head of pediatric surgery and later to be Surgeon General. I thought Dr. Koop was one of the most macho men I had ever met and sensed that no matter who was selected as Physician-in-Chief, he would dominate Philadelphia Children's Hospital. The atmosphere during my visit there was decidedly cool and I had the strong impression that I was the token woman whom they needed to fill the affirmative action rules for hiring new faculty members. In any event, the job was not suitable for me and I was not right for the search committee.

Next, I went to Case Western Reserve Medical School in Cleveland. I had acquaintances on the faculty and was warmly received. Case Western Reserve was noted for its work in infectious diseases and I knew it would be stimulating to work with the group there. I had interviews with numerous faculty members, including Dr. Charles Rammelkamp (affectionately known as Rammel) who was noted for his work on streptococcal infections and their relationship to rheumatic fever. Throughout the years I had been in awe of him at meetings of the Infectious Diseases Society, but our interview was really fun. He was a great raconteur and quickly put me at ease with some of his funny stories about his adventures in studying infectious diseases in foreign countries.

After meeting with a number of other faculty members, I was interviewed by Dr. Fred Robbins, Dean of the medical school and a Nobel laureate for his research on polio. He was quiet, almost shy, and perhaps the most modest scientist I have ever known, although he was one of the "greats" in the American Pediatric Society. He, too, put me at ease and the interview was a pleasant experience. I appreciated his courtesy and soon would have reason to appreciate it even more.

The night after the interviews, the chairman of the search committee and his wife gave a dinner for me at their home and Dr. Robbins proved to be the ultimate gentleman when I did one of the most embarrassing things of my life. The hostess served a beautiful dinner and was talking with Dr. Robbins, seated on her left, when she stopped in mid sentence. She looked at me while I spooned what I thought was the salad dressing onto my salad, and then, in a choked voice said, "Excuse me, Dr. Yow, but that is the sauce for the meat." I didn't even have time to respond before I heard Dr. Robbins say, "Oh, but that looks so delicious that I think I'll try it on my salad," whereupon he put a generous amount on his salad. What aplomb! What *savoir faire*! In later years, Fred Robbins was responsible for my being offered many opportunities in medicine, but the thing I appreciate most of all was his rescuing me so quickly from that awkward social situation.

The next day when I was offered an attractive position at Case Western Reserve, I asked for a short time to think it over, saying that there was one other school I had to visit before making a decision. The other was the medical school in San Antonio, a branch of the University of Texas system. Shortly after returning from Cleveland, I went for interviews in San Antonio where I was offered the chairmanship of the Department of Pediatrics. The position was also very appealing. Now I must make a choice.

I got into my car and drove up to the hill country of Texas to consider the two options. The more I looked at that rugged, beautiful country, the more I knew that I didn't want to leave Texas. I had about fifteen years more before retirement and I wanted to stay in Texas where I planned to live after retirement.

So back I went to Houston, notified the search committee at Case Western Reserve that I couldn't accept the position there, and then went to see Dr. Blattner to tell him that I was strongly considering moving to San Antonio. He seemed surprised but relieved. He said, "It's a good idea, because you really don't have any future here." I know he meant there was no administrative position at Baylor to which I could aspire, but I would have welcomed a comment like, "Well, I know you'll do a good job."

My decision about leaving Baylor and Houston was complicated by another very pleasant factor. While I was doing all this traveling about looking at jobs during the winter and spring of 1974, I had met Bob Roessler, a handsome professor of psychiatry who had come to Baylor from the University of Wisconsin, and he and I were becoming seriously interested in each other. Actually Bob and I had met the previous year but, on that occasion, I was so obnoxious that he avoided me for months. In fact, both of us acted in totally uncharacteristic ways. One day at lunch time Bob came into the faculty dining room and sat down at a table where I was sitting with several other faculty members. We were having a spirited discussion about remodeling and building houses and I was talking about the new house I had just built. Feeling that Bob was being excluded and wanting to have good manners, I turned to him and asked, "Where do you live?" With that he launched into a long discussion saying that he was divorced and was living in a small apartment. It was much later that I learned that he was a very quiet, self contained person who virtually never discussed his business in a situation like this, but he was so upset about living in reduced circumstances that he felt that he needed to explain. I, on the other hand, was so leery of any possible involvement that when I heard he was eligible, I lost all concern for his feelings or for good manners and responded in a biting tone, "I didn't ask for your life story, I just asked where you live!" After that encounter we avoided each other. Later he told me he vowed never to sit with that crazy woman again.

Eventually, though, he joined Ina, a woman psychiatrist friend of his, and me at lunch when we three women were laughing and obviously having a good time. I was telling the others about a movie with a South Carolina setting and saying that it was so good that I wouldn't mind seeing it again. When I left the table to go back to work, Bob followed me out to the elevator and asked me whether I would like to see the movie with him. Again, I had little charm. I answered that the movie was sentimental and that he probably wouldn't like it. He countered with, "Well, I'm sentimental," and with that, we agreed to go to see *Conrack*, an adaptation of Pat Conroy's book, *The River Is Wide.* Other couples have their songs; Bob and I have our movie.

Bob and I began to go out together very cautiously. He was recovering from his divorce and I from a recent love affair. Neither of us had marriage in mind. He was interested in my job search and put me on planes and met me at the airport when I returned.

Despite our cautious approach, Bob's and my courtship accelerated – although we had a difficult time finding any privacy. My grown children seemed to be omnipresent and my nephew, a medical student, was spending the spring with me, rooming on the balcony that overlooked the living room. Every time Bob said anything tender to me as we sat on the sofa below, we could hear offstage remarks from my nephew. We couldn't even court outside in the circular drive because the Chairman of Internal Medicine at Baylor lived on one side and a professor of Surgery lived on the other – both were quite conservative. We were thoroughly chaperoned!

Meanwhile, time for making a decision about moving to San Antonio was running out. It was May and the position in San Antonio needed to be filled by July, so I had to give the medical school an answer. On a Friday in the middle of May, I notified the dean that I would give him a definite answer on the following Monday.

Bob and I had plans to go to a party on Saturday night. On Friday night I had a premonition that he was going to propose to me on Saturday night. I paced the floor and spent a sleepless night. I hoped he would because I was in love with him, but I hoped he wouldn't so that I wouldn't have to make a decision about getting married. The next day, my daughter, Catherine, was taking bets on whether I would say "yes" and stay in Houston or "no" and go to San Antonio. She wouldn't say how she herself was betting. Sure enough, Bob called about noon on Saturday to ask whether he could come over early before the party. At 5 o'clock, he appeared at the door with roses in one hand and champagne in the other. We went into my study where we had a modicum of privacy and he asked me to marry him. Until that moment I had not known how I would react, but I didn't have to think. It felt right, and I just said, "Yes." He told me he had not wanted to ask me so soon, that he felt we needed to know each other better, but that he knew if he waited I would be gone and he didn't want to leave Baylor to be with me elsewhere.

So back I went to Dr. Blattner to tell him I had changed my mind, that I was staying at Baylor and marrying Bob Roessler. He knew Bob but he didn't know we were dating, and in his shock he blurted out, "That cultured man?" The term has become a family joke, because in July, five months after I met Bob for the second time, I married that "cultured man."

Another family joke resulted from my sister Catherine's thinly disguised disapproval of my marrying a Yankee. Bob was from Wisconsin, and although Catherine had not met Bob, she was apparently upset because he was from above the Mason-Dixon line. The degree of her concern became evident in a telephone conversation shortly after we were married. Early one morning my sister called.

"Martha, how are you? Were you asleep? This is the only time I can catch you."

"Well, yes I was asleep," I said, "but that's all right, I have to go to work soon, anyway. By the way, we really enjoyed your last letter about South Carolina's having it's first Republican governor in a hundred years. It was so funny!"

Her response came in frigid tones, "What was so funny about it? You just tell that Robert Roessler that if he thinks it's so funny, he should have been here during reconstruction days. Everybody knows that Republicans are nothing but alcoholics and carpet baggers!"

When I hung up, Bob asked, "What was that all about?" When I told him, he continued, "Was Catherine there during reconstruction days?" I explained that few southerners have ever gotten over the angst of reconstruction days. I am happy to report, however, that as time went on Catherine and Bob became friends, although we narrowly averted another misunderstanding.

Sometime later when we were planning a trip to visit my sister and her husband, Rhett, Bob said naively, "I'll enjoy being with Rhett. Since I am a Civil War buff, we can have a good time discussing it." My response was quick and vehement, "Oh no, Bob, please, no." My Yankee husband was finding that there's a lot to learn about living with a Southerner.

However, this time in my marriage there was no problem in balancing work and home life. I was established in my profession and there were no children to be considered. Bob and I had adequate domestic help and we shared the cooking. Of course, all was not sweetness and light in the marriage of two fifty-two year olds who were accustomed to being in control of things and who were temperamentally quite different. Bob was reserved and calm, and I was outgoing and impulsive. Our friends had misgivings about us, and we did have to do a lot of adapting, but eventually our personalities became complementary. Bob had what I thought of as a "listening heart." He was wonderfully understanding and supportive. And what did I bring to the union? Fun, I think.

Chapter 14

Another Bacterium Shapes My Career

Now that I was staying in Houston, my work went on as usual; but as always seemed to happen, my life was taken over by a new bacterium that shifted the direction of my research. It was not really a new bacterium, but one that in the 1970s became newly important as the leading bacterial infection in young infants – group B streptococcus (GBS). This streptococcus is related to the common group A streptococcus that causes strep throat. This organism, however, is a natural inhabitant of the vagina and the urethra, and ordinarily is carried silently and only rarely causes disease in adults. But a young infant who passes through a vagina harboring these organisms becomes heavily colonized with GBS and is at great risk for serious illness. Beginning in 1967, Ina had begun to see pneumonia and meningitis due to this organism in increasing numbers of newborn infants in the J.D. nursery, and as infectious disease consultant, I participated in their diagnosis and management. An invitation to speak at the University of Minnesota stimulated me to assess the magnitude of the problem so that I could present the material in my talk. The talk was to be a part of a day-long program honoring Dr. Wesley Spink who had been Ellard's mentor at the University of Minnesota. I was to represent Ellard and wanted to do an outstanding job.

In part, I was showing off because when we were in Minnesota I felt that the infectious disease group looked down their noses at my training and I remembered what a mistake they thought we were making by moving to Houston. In reality, after Ellard died and I began to succeed in academic medicine, Dr. Spink adopted me as a substitute for Ellard and was warm and encouraging. On this occasion, though, I felt that I had to prove something and undertook an enormous task. I hired my daughter and my niece and the three of us worked in the hospital record room many nights until midnight finding and reviewing the 122 cases of bacterial meningitis that had occurred in the 64,528 live births at J.D. from 1967 through 1974, so that I could try to define the importance of GBS. J.D. had one of the largest nurseries in the country and I still remember with great satisfaction the gasp of the Minnesota audience when I put up the slide showing these huge numbers. It was worth all the work in the catacomb-like J.D. record room.

Much of the credit should have gone to Ina, though, because the reconstruction of this story was in large part due to her powers of observation, her meticulous record keeping, her dedication to studying the interaction between paternal and infant infections, and her careful follow-up of sick infants. As was true of the Baylor rubella work, Ina provided the base in the nursery on which the rest of us could work.

This survey was the beginning of the clinical research on group B streptococcal infections that members of my section and I undertook. Indeed, it has continued for two decades and has become the life work of one of the infectious disease fellows, Dr. Carol Baker. Carol carried out careful bacteriologic work in my lab at Baylor, then spent a period of time at the Rockefeller Institute and two years at Harvard studying the immuno-chemistry of the group B streptococcus so that she could pursue preventive measures, such as the development of a vaccine. She has pursued this work for over twenty years and is now the leading world authority on group B streptococcal disease.

My interests led me in a different direction. I began to investigate transmission of the organism from pregnant women to their babies and to look for ways to prevent this transmission. Now I entered a fascinating type of clinical research with the obstetricians at Woman's Hospital of Texas, who helped me work with their patients. Group B streptococcus is sexually transmitted so that the logical approach to prevention had to include working with both husbands and wives. I enjoyed meeting with these young adults, trying new treatment regimens, and following the mothers and their infants through the delivery and for two months after delivery. An obstetrical hospital is a happy place, because most pregnancies result in well babies and the parents and grandparents are full of joy.

I had little money to carry out this work, that is, to pay an assistant, so my fellows and I did the work ourselves and it was fun. That is, we did the work with the parents and babies, and Ed Mason did the laboratory portion of the study. For months, we tried methods others had tried, such as treating mothers and fathers who carried the organism before delivery in an effort to have the mothers free of group B strep when they delivered, so they would not pass it to the babies during the birth process. This method proved to be impractical and ineffective, so I thought long thoughts about how I could insure that the mother's vagina was free of group B strep when the baby was born. Finally I thought, "Why not identify the mothers who harbored the organism several weeks before delivery and treat them as soon as they went into labor and during labor?" I hoped to get the appropriate antibiotic, ampicillin, into the amniotic fluid and also to eradicate the streptococcus from the vagina so that the infant could have a safe passage into the world.

Assessment of this approach required my being on call day and night so that I could obtain specimens from the mother as soon as she was admitted to the hospital in labor, and specimens during labor and after delivery, and serial specimens from the baby. The obstetricians worked out a method for collection of amniotic fluid without doing any invasive procedures that were not a part of the necessary obstetrical care. This fluid had to be kept cold until it was processed in the lab, so I spent many hours in the labor and delivery suite with an ice bucket full of test tubes, and I suspect I was something of a joke – a full professor running around day and night with specimens. But the results were so surprising and exciting that I didn't mind.

Bob, my husband, was really wonderful and supportive of

me in this endeavor. He too had conducted longitudinal studies and was something of a statistician. He knew how much work a study like this required and never resented the telephone ringing all hours of the day and night or my erratic hours. Each night at dinner, he asked me about the results, that is, how many women harbored the strep when they entered the labor suite and how many delivered infants who were colonized by the organism. The results were almost unbelievable – about two-thirds of the mothers who elected to be untreated but agreed to serve as controls passed organism to their infant, but none of the treated mothers did. Each day I expected to find that an infant of a treated mother would prove to have picked up the organism. As the numbers mounted, I held my breath until Ed Mason told me the culture results from each baby. As I told Bob about the results in protected infants as compared to the unprotected infants, he shared my excitement about the mounting statistical significance. With each delivery, I thought that surely there would be an infant in whom the treatment failed. But after we had twenty-six mother-infant pairs in each group – treated and untreated – the obstetricians, Ed, and I were able to report that treating a colonized mother during labor could prevent transmission of group B streptococcus to her infant. We did not prove that the infants would not pick up the organism later and develop disease, but we did show that the infant could be protected from acquiring the organism during labor and birth – the most critical time for an infant to be infected. This small, intense, precise study, published in the *Journal of the American Medical Association* in 1979 (Yow et al. 1979), led to the funding of a large study in Chicago that proved our method to be effective in preventing group B streptococcal disease the first week of life, the period when it is most dangerous. This method is now, in 1997, the standard of care advised by the American Academy of Pediatrics and the American College of Obstetrics and Gynecology. As I write this, I feel again the glow and excitement of having discovered a way to prevent this terrible disease in newborns, and I remember the fun of working with the obstetricians, nurses, and, most of all, with the happy parents.

* * * * * * * *

Dr. Blattner retired in 1977. He and I had certainly had our ups and downs, but I respected him for having built one of the largest and best pediatric departments and one of the finest children's hospitals in the nation. His successor was Dr. Ralph D. Feigin, a thirty-nine-year-old dynamo, whose subspecialty was infectious diseases. Our colleagues around the country watched with glee to see us lock horns. We disappointed them. During the first year of Ralph's tenure, I must admit that at times I felt competitive, but I helped him get his research started at Texas Children's Hospital, and he treated me with the utmost respect and consideration, including giving me a big raise. He had no prejudice against women – he respected performance!

* * * * * * * *

When I reached my late fifties, I was experiencing career burnout and felt a need for renewal. I had been working extremely hard for twenty-five years – seeing a tremendous number of patients, teaching, carrying out clinical research (always struggling for funds), being responsible for the overall financing and functioning of a large infectious disease service, traveling as a part of service on national committees – in other words, shouldering the responsibilities of any academician who heads a section, division, or even a small department. All of this intense activity began to take its toll. I developed acute, inflammatory arthritis in my hips, knees, and ankles and symptoms of a gastric ulcer. For a short time I made rounds in a wheel chair being pushed by the residents or fellows. Finally, Ed Ory, my doctor, hospitalized me for a thorough evaluation and, I suspect for an enforced rest.

When the results of the tests were in, Ed sat down in my hospital room and discussed the situation with me. He said, "Your blood tests indicate that you have some type of auto-immune arthritis similar to that of lupus, but a lot of your problems are due to stress. You either have to change your personality or your job. I have known you a long time and I don't think you can change your personality, so it will have to be your job."

I took his advice seriously. First I gave up my work for the American Academy of Pediatrics, work I loved, but work that required extensive traveling, often in severe winter weather. Next I notified the younger members of the infectious disease service that I would no longer rotate with them in running the service on nights and weekends. Many of the other section heads had already turned this over to younger faculty members. All of the infectious disease services at our teaching hospitals (Ben Taub, TCH, and the nursery at J.D.) were enormous and covering them took a lot of stamina – the stamina of younger doctors. My group B strep work at Woman's Hospital was at a good stopping place, and Carol Baker would carry on and extend this research.

Although I was beginning to give up the reins voluntarily, I was feeling somewhat disenfranchised, but within a few months I was improving physically. The swelling, heat, and pain in my joints began to recede, as did the ulcer symptoms, but emotionally I was somewhat "low in my mind."

I had, of course, heard the saying, "When God shuts the door, he opens a window," and that was exactly what happened to me. One day when I was sitting in my office, idly glancing over an NIH bulletin, my eye fell upon the announcement that senior investigator awards were being offered. These competitive awards provided a stipend for a one-year fellowship for established older investigators who agreed to pay back the award by working at least one year in an academic institution, after completion of the fellowship.

The opportunity seemed tailor-made for me. Who could be more senior? I was almost sixty. And, of course, the pay back was no problem. I planned to work at Baylor, not one, but many more years. The stipend was only half of my usual salary but I could settle for that.

I had never lost my interest in congenital CMV infections and, in fact, had done a few simple studies of this complex problem in the years since I had missed the opportunity to work with Dr. Weller at Harvard. I knew that Dr. Weller was no longer working with CMV but one of his trainees, Dr. Charles Alford, was conducting a large scale investigation of congenital CMV at the University of Alabama in Birmingham. When I called Dr. Weller to ask his opinion, he advised me to work with Dr. Alford if possible.

That night I discussed the matter with Bob, hoping that he

would approve of my applying for the fellowship. I told him that there was a non-stop flight between Houston and Birmingham and that I could come home at least once a month and for holidays. He was not thrilled over the prospect of my being away but, as usual, he was understanding. When I thanked him, he said, "What choice do I have? You really need a change." He was aware that twenty-five years is a long time for a person in academic medicine to stay at one school without a respite. He, himself had been on the faculty of three medical schools (The University of Rochester, The University of Wisconsin, and Baylor). He recognized the need of educational renewal for professors.

Dr. Alford agreed to be my mentor and this time, my chairman, Dr. Feigin, and Dr. William Butler, the President of Baylor, approved my application. Dr. Feigin even offered to supplement the stipend so that I would not have to make a financial sacrifice. I submitted my application to the NIH in January for the fellowship to begin in July. Months went by, July came and went and I dismissed the idea of going to Alabama but I wasn't very troubled about not getting the award because I was ambivalent about being away from Bob. Then in August I was surprised by receiving notification of a fellowship award to begin in September.

Bob helped me rush around and late in August drove with me to Birmingham to help me move into a small apartment. I felt terribly lonely when he left, but was thrilled about studying CMV infections in mothers and their infants and about learning how to conduct some worthwhile CMV research when I returned to Baylor.

Charlie's laboratory proved to be the ideal choice for my sabbatical. It's purpose was the study of congenital and perinatal infections (herpes, chlamydia, CMV) with the main emphasis on CMV, and I was surrounded by individuals who were intensely involved in providing new knowledge about these serious diseases. There were five faculty members – Charlie Alford, Sergio Stagno, Rich Whitley, Bob Pass, and Fred Lakeman; two fellows – Meyer Dworsky and Paul Griffiths; a laboratory supervisor – Rolph Reynolds; and three technicians. To my surprise, the faculty members spent most of their time in the laboratory. At that time Charlie had no clinical responsibilities and the other faculty members had remarkably light assignments in patient care and teaching, compared to the norm at Baylor. No wonder this group had such an active, productive research record.

The laboratory itself was equally amazing – several thousands of square feet equipped with laboratory benches, virology hoods, microscopes of various types, a walk-in incubator (mine in Houston was a small table model), walk-in refrigerator and a walk-in freezer. I was given a small cubicle with a lab bench for a desk and a window that I would grow to love when, in the early winter twilights, I watched the city lights come on. It was too good to be true. I felt as if I had come into the land of plenty!

The first morning when I reported to work I was excited but apprehensive about my lack of laboratory skills. I had supervised bacteriology technicians for years but had not actually sat at the bench handling specimens, test tubes, or pipettes for at least twenty years. I was concerned about my lack of manual dexterity but, after all, I was there to learn laboratory techniques so that I could teach a technician when I returned to Baylor.

My apprehension was nothing compared to that of the twenty-seven-year-old, second-year fellow, Meyer Dworsky, who was assigned to supervise a sixty-year-old woman professor. He was somewhat in awe of me, because I had been chairman of the Redbook Committee of The American Academy of Pediatrics, but the awe didn't last long when he saw how inept I was at the bench and soon he began to address me affectionately as "Most Distinguished Professor." Meyer was a no-nonsense person and he was determined that I would do things right, especially since I would be working on a project with him and might ruin valuable specimens that he had spent hours collecting. Rolph Reynolds, the laboratory supervisor, was an expert teacher and he, too, was tough. One day when I protested that I could not hold test tube stoppers with my left, little finger, as he had told me to do, he countered, "If you can't do that you can't do virology." I practiced until I learned to do it

Charlie Alford was the most perfectionistic of all. Charlie was about fifteen years younger than I. We had been acquaintances for a number of years, but now as he welcomed me into his group, our relationship had changed. There was no question of who was in charge. He was the professor and I was the first-year fellow who was going to do things right. I recognized the appropriateness of this and became the instant student.

When Charlie outlined my project for the year, in my naivete, I thought, "Oh great. I can do that." Ignorance really is bliss! It wasn't long before I began to think that, "the new kid on the block" had been given an assignment that the others were avoiding. I was to work with breast milk, isolating CMV and determining whether the breast milk contained any immune substances that would neutralize the virus. Breast milk was hard to work with, but Sergio Stagno had worked out the method and I learned to culture the milk fairly quickly. The search for immune substances was a different matter. After I so glibly said that I would glad to do the project, I found out that the other fellows and technicians were choking back their laughter at my enthusiasm because they knew what a tough assignment I had fallen heir to.

The technicians warned me that neutralization, the technique used to detect any immune substances, was fairly difficult using blood and with breast milk would be even more difficult. They told me, too, that the long, laborious work of looking at the neutralization tests under the microscope would make me nauseated. I dismissed the latter comment because I couldn't see how looking through a microscope could make one nauseated.

I found out that the naysayers were right on both points. My neutralization tests were tedious and time consuming and often had to be repeated. I worked all day on Mondays setting up the neutralization plates that contained the breast milk specimens and put them in the walk-in incubator on my own shelf. (Each of us had a shelf with our name on it. Much to Charlie's consternation, I labeled mine, "Texas Back Forty." He was dignified and didn't always like my irreverent humor.) On Thursdays I examined the plates under the microscope. Often the tests had failed. On Thursday nights, I would call Bob to tell him how discouraged I was or he would call me to ask how the week's tests had gone. He was wonderfully comforting and always expressed confidence that soon I would master the technique.

The times the tests worked were gratifying, but not pure unsullied joy, because reading them did cause nausea, probably the result of moving the plates back and forth to read them under the microscope. Somehow it disturbed one's vestibular nerve and all of a sudden, it produced severe nausea with retching, just like sea sickness. When this happened, the only cure was to get up, walk around and wait until the nausea subsided. Eventually I mastered the technique so that my tests were successful but the attacks of nausea continued and, to this day, I can't stand the smell of the reagents we used.

After a few weeks, during which everybody in the lab became aware of my willingness to work hard and my intense desire to learn, I became a real part of the group and we could laugh at each other's foibles. And, of course, the person we focused on the most was the boss, Charlie, although we had enormous respect for him. It was a real role reversal for me – being a part of the group who enjoyed moments of upmanship on the leader, rather than being the leader who was on the receiving end.

Charlie's office was outside of the lab and he spent most of his time there, writing grants, papers, or chapters. But he wanted to be aware of everything going on in the lab, so each day he paced though the lab, sometimes several times a day. He was a real pacer, back and forth wandering in and out of every cubicle, looking over our shoulders, observing our work, and reading our lab notes. Usually there was a good deal of laughter and conversation in the lab, but a sudden silence in the front part of the lab alerted us to his visits during which all was quiet.

When I had been there about a month, Charlie went into my cubicle while I was in the lab and examined my log book where all my experiments were recorded. He came out very concerned, "You aren't keeping your log book right. I want you to get a calendar and record what you are scheduled to do each day. For example, 'Change the medium in tubes A-27 through A-45' or, 'Split the cells in bottles B-4 and B-5.'" He glared around the lab and announced loudly "Martha, you aren't being taught right. I'll just have to teach you myself." Of course, Meyer, the lab supervisor, and the technicians continued to teach me, but many days Charlie sat side by side with me while I was working with specimens under the virology hood or examining results in the small, dark microscope rooms.

My colleagues got great glee out of my tutelage by Charlie, because they knew how demanding he was and because they thought that some of his methods were outdated, but I liked it. Charlie taught me CMV laboratory techniques from the ground up. He taught me the things that Dr. Weller had taught him. Sometimes I heard others in the lab whisper, "obsolete, obsolete," but what I learned from Charlie was meticulous attention to detail and none of it was obsolete. I appreciated his interest and knew that he was teaching me valuable basic principles, but I couldn't resist being a bit mischievous. Knowing that Charlie would be reading my calendar, I inserted little things like "Play golf on Tuesday," "Lunch with the girls on Thursday," or "Leave for Florida on Friday," none of which I planned to do, of course. But, despite my clowning around, and the misgivings of the lab staff, Charlie and I enjoyed our work sessions.

Things didn't always go smoothly, however. Inevitably we had small clashes. One morning before Charlie came in everything had gone wrong. Rolph Reynolds had reproached me about something to do with my disposal bucket, Meyer gave me one of his, "Most Distinguished Professor" reprimands because I had made a mistake with one of his specimens. Then Charlie walked up beside me when I was doing something tedious under the hood, demanding "Why are you using expensive bottles instead of test tubes?" I blew, "Because I want to!" He turned on his heel and stalked out of the lab, shouting over his shoulder, "It's a good thing you are already a full professor because you'd never get to be one here." A terrible hush fell over the lab. Everyone was appalled by the clash of the two professors, but since neither of us harbored grudges, the rift was quickly healed. After all, how could I be upset when I was having such a valuable learning experience?

My life outside of the lab was wonderful, too. Birmingham was a beautiful place. I had thought that it would be a smoky, industrial city, but by the time I arrived in 1980, the steel mills had been closed for a number of years, the downtown district was being improved, and the residential areas were the most beautiful I had ever seen anywhere. Each morning I drove slowly down winding roads through lush colorful growth surrounding spacious homes. There were hundreds of dogwood trees in the fall with brilliant red leaves, chrysanthemums, and other fall flowers. In the spring, the trees were festooned with purple wisteria and now the dogwood trees were covered with white blossoms and gardens were full of daffodils and azaleas. Each day I took time to "smell the roses." I arrived at work happy and bursting with energy. Never since I had been in high school had I felt so carefree. I was like a kid let out of school for summer vacation.

My social life was full and eclectic with good times with Meyer and his wife and Paul Griffiths, an advanced fellow from London, and his wife, both of whom had a dry British sense of humor, and the faculty members and their wives. Mary Elizabeth, Charlie's wife, was especially welcoming to me and we soon became good friends. Also I discovered southern cousins in Birmingham. What Southerner can go anywhere in the deep south without running into relatives?

My friendship with the three young women technicians was especially fun. We frequently had dinner together where I heard about their boy friends or their ambitions. Too, they inveigled me into playing racquet ball. Yes, racket ball! I thought tennis a much better choice for me, but they wanted to play racquet ball, so we did. I was a little worried about it, thinking, "If I break my leg, how will I ever be able to explain to Dr. Feigin, my chairman, or to Bob how I could break my leg on a sabbatical?"

I made frequent trips to Texas, one of which was especially notable. My second grandchild, Katy, was born in San Antonio. She caused quite a stir in the Alabama laboratory and gave me a terrible fright. When my son, Ellard, called me to tell me that she had arrived he said, "She's very small, Mother. She weighs about three and a half pounds." Three and a half in a full term baby! I was terribly concerned. The first thing that all of us in the CMV lab thought about was a congenital infection. I was on the next plane west, armed with test tubes to transport specimens back to Alabama. Before I left Alabama, though, I was on the phone talking to Ina. She arranged for a neonatologist from the University of Texas medical school in San Antonio to see Katy. When I arrived, I saw a pitifully thin infant who captured my heart instantly. I was deeply troubled by her appearance, but the consulting pediatrician reassured me. He said he found nothing wrong with her, but marked undernutrition and that since she was doing well and breast feeding vigorously, he thought that she should stay in the newborn nursery for a period of several weeks during which her mother would come in and breast feed her at frequent intervals. He was right. She was just starved probably from placental insufficiency and now that she was in the outside world, she gained very rapidly. After a few days in which I reassured myself and my son and his wife, I collected specimens and returned to Birmingham. All of us in the Birmingham lab breathed a deep sigh of relief when the tests were negative! Katy was born in November and by January she was a fat, healthy baby. Today, as I write this, she is a stunningly beautiful fifteen year old.

With all of these interesting activities, the twelve months of my sabbatical sped by and soon I was heading home to Houston and Bob, refreshed and with all bones intact.

* * * * * * * *

Back at Baylor I resumed my clinical and teaching duties and began to look for laboratory space where I could start a CMV research project. (Before leaving for the year in Birmingham, I had given my lab space at Baylor to Dr. Carol Baker for her group B strep research, and even if I still had the space, I had no money for virologic equipment.) I hoped that the pathology department at Texas Children's Hospital would let me start a much needed virus diagnostic laboratory there. I would be glad to direct it in exchange for space and equipment to initiate a CMV research program. The head of pathology recognized the need, but there was no available space.

After a good deal of unsuccessful searching, I went to see Dr. Vernon Knight, Chairman of the Department of Microbiology at Baylor, and after hearing my dilemma, he offered me the position of the Director of The Virus Diagnostic Laboratory at Methodist Hospital, a laboratory he had established and directed for many years. In exchange for my work, the hospital would pay a portion of my salary, provide the necessary equipment, and give me a small space where a research technician, an infectious disease fellow, and I could work.

I managed to get small grants to pay a fellow and a technician from The March Of Dimes and several other granting agencies and worked out an arrangement with the Woman's Hospital (where I had done the group B strep work) to pay me a small fee for testing every newborn in its nursery for CMV infection. Since this amounted to about 2500 specimens per year, it was my major source of research support. Again, generous Houston women helped me. Dr. Najia White wanted to work part time and volunteered her services, a few wealthy Houston women gave me funds to establish the program, and two prominent Houston women worked with me collecting specimens and interviewing parents.

Creakingly, the program got off the ground in 1981. With the help of Dr. Larry Taber, my long-standing friend and colleague in infectious diseases, and with the addition of Dr. Gail Demmler, an outstanding infectious disease fellow and later a faculty member, I began to build a strong CMV research unit. Within a few years, we outgrew the space in the Methodist Hospital Laboratory, and once again, Dr. Knight came to my rescue by giving me lab space in the Department of Microbiology.

Why did I feel that the study of congenital CMV was so important? Few people had ever heard of it and most doctors didn't understand it, but it was the leading infectious cause of mental retardation and deafness. Each year in the United States, year in and year out, an estimated forty thousand infants were born infected with CMV, as shown by the presence of virus in the their urine and saliva. Four thousand of these infants showed signs of the infection at birth, including small size, small heads, enlarged livers and spleens, anemia, bleeding problems, involvement of the eyes, and cerebral palsy. Ten percent, or 4 thousand of these children died in infancy. The other 36 thousand had no symptoms at birth, but of these, 4 to 8 thousand would later be found to be deaf or to have neurologic problems. In 1971, Dr. Weller, in a landmark article in *The New England Journal of Medicine*, had alerted us to the problems of congenital CMV disease stating that, "This problem causes inestimable human suffering and costs the nation more than $1.8 billion a year" (Weller 1971). Despite his warning, the same situation still existed in 1981, and in the ten years after the publication of his article another 4 hundred thousand of our nation's children had been born with congenital CMV infection, of whom 40 to 80 thousand would have significant problems. This was a major public health dilemma and preventive measures were urgently needed.

When we began our work in Houston in 1981, what did we want to learn and what did we hope to contribute? Overall, of course, our goal was to join other scientists in adding knowledge that would lead to prevention of CMV infection in mothers and their newborn infants. Before this could be accomplished, however, there were many questions that had to be answered. Was the incidence of congenital infection the same all over the United States? Were there factors (age, race, socioeconomic status) that put certain women of childbearing age more at risk for infection than others? How did the mothers acquire the virus (from their husbands or from young children)? How did it spread within the family? If mothers had experienced the infection before pregnancy, would their immunity protect their offspring? The answer to the latter question was particularly important in considering the potential usefulness of a vaccine. Were there other practical methods to prevent women from acquiring the infection during pregnancy?

In addition to learning more about maternal infection, we needed to know more about the outcome of their infected infants, especially those who had no obvious signs of problems at birth. Here, Ina would be an essential member of the CMV research team. For many years, she had been conducting follow-up studies of newborn infants with problems, such as genetic defects, infection, prematurity, and damage due to maternal drug abuse, and was expert in this type of research. Following the rubella epidemic, she and I had worked with a small number of CMV-infected infants for many years before my sabbatical. Now we were in a really good situation to work together again. I would work with the obstetricians at Woman's Hospital studying CMV in pregnant women and detecting the congenitally infected infants in the 2,500-3,000 newborns delivered there annually. Ina, who was now head of the developmental pediatrics section, would evaluate and arrange care for these infants. She would follow their progress for a long period, hopefully through early school years.

A great deal was known about the infants who were symptomatic at birth, but we were particularly concerned about those who were born shedding the virus in their urine, but had no obvious signs and symptoms. Many people, including doctors, asked why it was important to detect these children and to follow them so closely since there was no treatment for CMV infection. But all of us involved in CMV research were acutely aware of how detrimental undiagnosed deafness or neurologic problems were and still are to young children. Often they suffer severe psychologic damage by being considered obstinate or retarded; thus early detection is necessary so that remedial care begin at the youngest age possible.

Both Ina and I were excited about working together again. Of course, we would have to struggle for financial support, but we figured, "there was a dance in the old dames yet." Ina called us "survivors." Bob said, "No, you're fighters."

* * * * * * * *

And struggle and survive we did. Our study at Woman's Hospital, involving almost five thousand women and their infants, answered many of our questions. Our results showed that the incidence of congenital infection was the same in Houston as that in Birmingham, and suggested that it was probably the same throughout the United States. Our results also agreed with the findings of the Alabama group that age, race, and socioeconomic factors put certain women at increased risk of becoming infected and transmitting the virus to their infants. Two groups of women were most likely to become infected by CMV during pregnancy – young women who were poor and non-white and older white women from a more privileged economic bracket. Our study also added proof that maternal immunity (from an infection prior to pregnancy) protected the fetus or modified the damage. This finding indicated that a vaccine would be valuable in preventing severe congenital CMV infection and told us that the vaccine strategy might well be administration of the vaccine in the preteen or early teenage years.

Larry Taber had a vast amount of data and serial blood specimens collected in an intense ten-year study. He was able to clarify the pattern of infection throughout childhood and the spread within families. Although it could spread between husbands and wives, young children were the most common source of infection to mothers.

Gail Demmler developed rapid diagnostic laboratory techniques and added important information about occupational risks, or lack of risks, within hospital settings where careful hand washing and other practices were followed. But during this time, Dr. Robert Pass at the University of Alabama was finding that there was an added risk to workers in day-care centers where large numbers of young children were shedding the virus, and hygienic practices were sometimes less stringent.

While we were waiting for the development of an effective, safe vaccine, Gail began investigating other methods of protecting non-immune women of child-bearing age from the virus. She showed that avoidance of contact with the urine and saliva of infected children could protect women from infection. She spent a great deal of time counseling mothers about how to protect themselves, such as not allowing a child to drink from one's glass or share a spoon, as a mother might do in cajoling a child to eat. She realized that it was important for mothers to be able to express affection for their children, but she suggested that mothers avoid kissing a child on a saliva-wet face – substituting a kiss on top of the head or hugging. One thing she advised that most surprised me was, "Don't share a toothbrush with your child." I had never known that people shared toothbrushes with their children, but she assured me that some parents did indeed do so in teaching their toddlers to brush their own teeth. This study was extremely time consuming, but Gail was able to show that mothers who observed these simple hygienic precautions did not become infected, whereas some of the mothers who elected not to use the precautions, but agreed to serve as controls, did become infected.

Meanwhile, Ina and her colleagues were learning more about congenitally infected infants – both those symptomatic at birth and those who were shedding virus at birth, but had no symptoms. Using new techniques, Ina and her group were able to test hearing function in newborn infants reliably. In their work, they also followed the development of these infants closely and rechecked their hearing at specified intervals. Their findings showed that deafness in some children progressed as they grew older.

Our research during these years answered many of our questions, and we had done it all in a small lab, on a minuscule budget, with the help of a lot of generous people. These were happy productive days in which we all shared a sense of pride.

Chapter 15

The Top of the Ladder

THE LAST DAY OF 1988 FOUND ME sitting in my office surrounded by packing boxes and filing cabinets. It was the last day of my thirty-three years as a Baylor faculty member and the last day of my duties as Editor of the *Journal of Infectious Diseases*. Today, I just let my thoughts drift as I swiveled around with my back to my lonely looking desk. I looked out at the view from my big window, high over Main Street and relaxed and reminisced as I enjoyed the huge Texas sky filled with giant cumulus clouds. The athletic field at Rice University was still green and was surrounded by the muted greens of Houston's live oaks. Still further away was the beautiful Transco Tower on the western horizon. On hundreds of afternoons I had luxuriated in this same scene, and I never tired of it and its changing moods–beautiful, mild sunny days like today, or days with misty overcast skies, or dramatic afternoons with menacing black clouds sweeping eastward and blotting out the view and suddenly pelting my window with the heavy rain of the subtropics. Best of all were the glorious sunsets with the sun sliding down the Transco tower turning it into shimmering gold from top to bottom. I loved the view, I loved my work, I loved Houston, and yet I was leaving.

So much had happened since my Sabbatical in Alabama. I

had given up my administrative responsibilities as chief of the Pediatric Infectious Disease Section. I really believed that twenty-five years in that role was long enough, and that a younger person with fresh ideas could do a better job. I had watched too many leaders hang on too long, overshadowing younger faculty members and blocking their progress. Somehow, it had always reminded me of a garden bed where the older plants were not removed and the young plants could not thrive. I was determined that I would not outstay my usefulness. My decision, however, was not completely altruistic. I was exercising considerable self interest, because I wanted to free up time for my CMV research.

But how in the world did I become an editor? My life always seemed to be full of surprises, never static and never dull. And this surprise was the best of all.

One day in the late spring of 1983, I was enduring the usual interminable wait at one of the Baylor elevators, and Dr. Robert Couch, a member of the infectious disease section in internal medicine, was waiting beside me. Almost as if on an impulse, he said, "Martha, Dr. George Jackson is resigning as Editor of *The Journal of Infectious Diseases,* and those of us on the editorial committee of the Society (of Infectious Diseases) are looking for a replacement. Your name came up as a possible candidate in the recent meeting, but I told the others that you're probably too busy, but that I would mention it to you. Are you interested?" I was almost too stunned to answer. *The Journal of Infectious Diseases* is the official publication of the Infectious Diseases Society of America and the most prestigious journal in the field of infectious diseases in the entire world. I had been a titular member of the editorial board of the *Journal* for five years, but had never been called on to do anything but review a few manuscripts. In fact, I had complained that I was not asked to review more. I finally stammered out, "Let me think about it, Bob. Maybe I can give up something else I'm doing."

Early the next morning I went to see Bob Couch to learn more particulars. He explained that the individual selected must have a significant amount of time to devote to the *Journal* and had to agree to serve a five-year term. There would, of course, be other candidates for the position, and the committee's decision would be influenced not only the individual's ability and commitment, but also, to a large degree, by the support of one's school in providing office space. Even more essential was the presence of a critical number of qualified scientists in the candidate's medical community to serve as associate editors. This group of associate editors must have the expertise to cover all aspects of infectious diseases (bacteriology, virology, mycology, immunology, epidemiology, and even statistics).

The rest of the day I ruminated over this information. Certainly the Texas Medical Center in Houston had a large number of infectious disease experts whose experiences covered every aspect of the field. I thought, too, that I would have Baylor's support, since Dr. William Butler, its president, was an infectious disease expert himself and would realize the prestige to be gained by having the *Journal* located at Baylor. There had been only two previous editors, Dr. Edward Kass at Harvard and Dr. George Jackson at the University of Illinois. It would be a real honor to have the editorial office of the *Journal of Infectious Diseases* at Baylor.

Questions were tumbling over in my mind. Could I do it? Did I have the ability? Could I learn to run a journal in such a short time (If elected, I would have to assume the helm within six months)? Which of my duties could I relinquish to free up at least half of my time? That last question was relatively easy to answer. I would resign as director of the Virus Diagnostic Laboratory at Methodist Hospital and I would give up seeing patients except those involved in my CMV research.

My greatest concern was how Bob would feel about my taking on this responsibility. He wanted both of us to retire in three years when we were sixty-five, and I had promised to do so. But the editorship was for a five-year term, and if Bob agreed, it would mean staying in Houston two years longer than we had planned.

That night I approached Bob with trepidation, but when he saw how much it meant to me, he unselfishly agreed to stay in Houston the additional years. So now I was free to pursue the matter.

After obtaining the support of Dr. Butler and my chairman, Dr. Feigin, also a leader in the field of infectious diseases, I submitted a proposal to the Editorial Committee of the Infectious Diseases Society. A few months later, I received a call from the president of the Society telling me that I was the new editor of the *Journal.*

Almost immediately I was off to the editorial office at the University of Illinois to arrange a smooth transition of the *Journal* to Baylor. After a briefing by Dr. George Jackson, I spent time at the University of Chicago Press, where the *Journal* was published. A major part of my job as editor would be interacting with the Press on business matters – something about which I knew absolutely nothing, but was determined to learn.

My next trip was to Boston to visit Dr. Edward Kass, who had started the *Journal* and had been its editor for the first ten years. He was the founder and editor of a second infectious diseases journal, *The Reviews of Infectious Diseases,* and maintained a busy editorial office. Ed gave me a warm welcome and offered many valuable suggestions. He then invited me to observe the workings of his editorial office and sit in on his monthly meeting of his editorial associates where manuscripts were discussed and selected for publication.

Best of all, knowing that I needed an assistant editor, Ed generously recommended a member of his own staff, Dr. Dale Spriggs. Dale was perfect for the position. He had learned the business from the bottom up. Not only did he know how to run an editorial office, interact with the printer, and teach copy editors, but he was also a molecular virologist and brought important scientific knowledge to our editorial group. To me, he brought his youthful optimism (he was in his late twenties), as he tutored me in new technology and shared his wonderful sense of humor. We became great friends!

There was no problem in assembling an impressive group of associate editors, because the Texas Medical Center was noted for its cadre of infectious disease experts, both at Baylor and at the adjacent University of Texas Health Science Center. With Dale's help, I recruited an office staff of bright young people. Now we were ready to go, but it was well into the fall of 1983, and our first issue was due January first. We went through some very anxious moments when I was not certain we could really produce that first issue. But we did, and during the next five years, we produced fifty-nine more issues.

I loved being an editor. Each afternoon, I read manuscripts and talked to authors and reviewers all over the nation and sometimes overseas. My life and my perspective expanded through this experience, because I got to know so many interesting people with widely divergent backgrounds. Some days, I talked with famous people who assumed we would give them almost unlimited space to publish their work. I disabused them of this idea as gently and diplomatically as I could. At an Infectious Diseases Society reception one evening, Albert Sabin said, "I don't know anyone who can say 'no' in such a charming manner as Martha Yow." Other days, I advised first-time, unknown authors how to improve their articles. They were so eager and receptive that it was fun working with them.

We received papers from all over the world, and, not infrequently, it was evident that scientists were conducting research under extremely difficult circumstances. Manuscripts from eastern Europe or from Third World countries were often poorly typed on coarse paper.

We were so accustomed to manuscripts typed double-spaced on pristine bond, that manuscripts which differed always attracted our attention.

We had an unusual experience working with a scientist from a remote province in China. His manuscript arrived on yellow paper so coarse that wooden chips were still present in it. His paper had scientific merit, but the English was so difficult to interpret that we could not revise it in a publishable form. The associate editors and I agreed that I should advise the author that we would reconsider his article if he obtained help from a writer whose first language was English. Many weeks later, he returned the manuscript, still typed on rough paper, but written in remarkably stilted, unusual English. His covering letter apologized for the delay, and explained that the only person he could find to help him was a Catholic priest. This time, Dale Spriggs and I improved his paper as much as possible and accepted it for publication. The readers must have wondered at the somewhat ecclesiastical writing style. That Chinese author sent me one of the most heart-warming thank-you letters I ever received and enclosed a beautiful collection of Chinese stamps. Yes, I loved being an editor!

I would be hard pressed to say which I had enjoyed most, our CMV research or being editor of the *Journal.* I only knew that the last years of my academic life had been full and happy, and that I had reached the top rung of my personal ladder. There were no more rungs that I wanted to climb. I was happy to be exactly where I was.

When I decided to retire, my friends and associates expressed concern that I couldn't be happy "doing nothing." I assured them that I wouldn't be doing nothing. Bob and I had chosen San Diego for our retirement because of its climate, its mountains and beaches, but also because I planned to work part-time at the medical school in San Diego as a volunteer. I had already collaborated on CMV research with one of the faculty members there and was in the process of organizing a CMV workshop at the Centers for Disease Control in Atlanta. I would continue to be active on national committees, but I would save plenty of time for golf and traveling with Bob. It was time for a new balancing act.

These long thoughts had brought the winter afternoon to a close, and as I turned the key in the door, I had some feelings of sadness at leaving, but mostly I felt that I was starting a new adventure, and I heard a little voice inside saying,

> before i m through
> you get me pet
> there s a dance or two
> in the old dame yet (Marquis 1927).

References

American Medical Association. 1991. *Women in medicine in America – In the mainstream.* Chicago IL: AMA.

Butler L. J., Yow, M.D., and J. B. Reinhart,1946. Meningitis due to Hemophilus influenzae. *N.C. Med J.* 7:8-12.

Marquis, D. archy and mehitabel. 1927. Garden City, NY: Doubleday & Co., Inc.

Melnick, J. L. 1988. Live attenuated polio vaccines. In *Vaccines*, edited by S. A. Plotkin and E. A. Mortimer, 115-157. Philadelphia: Harcourt Brace Jovanovich.

Rosenberg, R. 1992. *American women in the twentieth century.* New York: Hill & Wang - Noonday Press.

Rudolph, A. J., Yow, M.D., Phillips, A., Desmond, M.F., Blattner, R. J., and Melnick, J. L. 1965. Transplacental rubella infection in newly born infants. *JAMA* 191:843-845.

S.C. Const., art. XVII §3.

Weller, T. H. 1971. The cytomegalovirus: ubiquitous agents with protean clinical manifestations. *N. Engl. J. Med.* 285:203-214.

Worthington, W. C., Pratt-Thomas, H. R., and Sawyer, W. A. 1991. *The Medical University of South Carolina. A family album: men who made the Medical Center.* (The Medical University of South Carolina) Spartanburg SC: The Reprint Co.

Yow, M.D., Mason, E. O., Leeds, L. J., Thompson, P. K., Clark, D. J., and Gardner, S. E. 1979. Ampicillin prevents intrapartum transmission of group B streptococcus. JAMA 241:1245-1247.